SAY GOODBYE TO BACK PAIN

Overlooked Scientific Discoveries Reveal Powerful
New Solutions for Back Pain, Sciatica, and Stenosis
No Matter What Treatments Have Failed You Before.

Dr. Russell Horine DC

Dr. Natalie Horine DC, MS

Dr. Lee Horine DC, MS

ISBN: 1508623368
ISBN 13: 9781508623366
Library of Congress Control Number: 2015903192
CreateSpace Independent Publishing Platform
North Charleston, South Carolina

DEDICATION

This book is dedicated to our past, present, and future patients.

ACKNOWLEDGMENTS

We would like to take this opportunity to acknowledge Andrea Horine who has given her unyielding support and has tolerated countless late nights and early mornings listening to us discuss back pain research and new ideas. Without her as a loving mother and wife, this book would have never been a possibility.

We would also like to thank Dean Horine for his foundational work compiling and assessing the DICE protocol. Without his intensive labor this book would not have been nearly as rich.

Without great mentors to challenge and push us to accept nothing short of excellence this endeavor would never have occurred. Dr. Lee and Dr. Natalie would like to thank Dr. Marc Ellis, Dr. Paula Rhodes, and Dr. Keith Rau for their early and continued support and friendship. "You all taught us that learning never stops and mastery is an intangible quest that is worth the journey."

Intended Use and Disclaimer

The content within this book is intended to present and emphasize the prevalence of low back conditions while offering clinical suggestions and protocols on overall health maintenance.

The medical information within this book should not serve to diagnose, treat, cure, or prevent disease in anyway. The reader should always consult their health or medical professional before utilizing any of the suggestions contained herein.

It is also the absolute responsibility of the reader of this book to comply within all local and federal regulations regarding the use of such information as it relates to their type and scope of practice.

TABLE OF CONTENTS

PART II: THE CHRONIC STRESS CYCLE

PART III: STRATEGIES FOR REDUCING CHRONIC STRESS AT HOME AND WORK

INTRODUCTION

"Doctor, what's wrong with my back?
How did this happen to me?"

I was sitting across from Janet, a nurse at the local hospital. We were both looking at the MRI study of her back. She was in her mid-thirties and had always been a very active person—busy hiking, cycling, and playing tennis. And here she was looking at MRIs of her low back that showed significant disc degeneration in her lower spine. Disc degeneration is where the discs (pads between the spinal bones) break down and flatten out.

For the past year she had been suffering from back pain and sciatica. Sciatica is a condition in which nerve irritation causes shooting pain down the legs and sometimes past the ankles. Her symptoms started off gradually, and the pain was only occasional. She initially decreased her outdoor activities, assuming the symptoms would pass. Being athletic, she had strained her back before, but it had always gotten better given a little time. This was different.

Not only did the pain not go away, it continued to worsen until now she had a hard time just getting through her daily work at the hospital. She was taking painkillers, muscle relaxers, and anti-inflammatory medication. And just two weeks ago, she had been prescribed antidepressants because giving up the things she loved to do had caused her to become very depressed.

I remember this conversation well. It was in August of 2009, and it was the beginning of the turning point in my practice.

As we were going over the imaging studies, she had all the questions that most people in her situation have, and I was giving her the typical answers that doctors are trained to give when someone has a condition like this. It wasn't the first time I had found myself in this type of situation.

The problem was that I had become increasingly uncomfortable with my answers to these questions.

Don't get me wrong; I had treated thousands of patients with similar conditions in my previous thirty years of practice. I had built a reputation in my community as being very effective at treating low back conditions. It wasn't lack of confidence in my methods or treatments that made me uneasy with my answers. It was simply that the answers I (and most other health-care practitioners) gave didn't mesh with the recent research regarding low back conditions.

Over the years the patients were different, but the questions were the same.

"What caused this to happen?"

"Is it just normal aging?"

"What causes the pain to come and go?"

"It all started when I bent over to pick something up. How could that cause my disc to bulge?"

"When I get stressed out, it seems to get worse. Does that mean it's partly in my head?"

"I'm doing all the exercises my therapist recommended. At first it was helping, but now it's not helping at all. Why did it stop working?"

"I've tried everything—medication, injections, physical therapy, acupuncture, massage. They all helped for a little while, but the pain keeps coming back. Is surgery my only option?"

Now, in retrospect, here are a couple of questions that were not asked but that should be added to the list.

"As my back pain gets worse, I seem to have less energy and feel more depressed. Is it from the pain...or something else?"

"After the onset of back pain, my overall health has seemed to decline. Is there a connection?"

I never intended to write this book. But, after my experience with Janet, I decided to commit a few months of research to do a better job of answering these questions.

The deeper I dug, the more questions I had. This three-month, self-imposed research project grew into six months and then a year.

I became a little obsessed.

After two years of researching, I realized that my findings were evolving into a book, and I needed help.

At the time, my son and daughter-in-law were involved in graduate work at Life University, a top-tier chiropractic research university. They were both working to integrate chiropractic, functional neurology, and kinesiology.

I needed their trained minds to help put the pieces together for me. With their broad experience in multiple fields of study, as well as their hands-on experience of working with extremely complex conditions, I thought they would be the perfect fit.

When I discussed my initial findings with them, they were intrigued, and I was able to convince them to jump on board. This was the true beginning of this book.

We thought the book would take another year to write, but soon it had turned into three.

The project took longer than we thought, but the upside of this was that Dr. Natalie and Dr. Lee became so excited about the discoveries we were making that they decided to join my practice and help implement and fine-tune our new procedures.

My initial quest to answer a dozen questions had opened up a Pandora's box. The benefit that I was not expecting was that, by answering these questions, we fundamentally changed the way we assess and treat low back pain in our clinic.

As you will learn, the traditional treatments of chronic low back pain, disc degeneration, and sciatica do not have near the success rate that they should. This is not merely my opinion but is based on current statistics.

My hope is that by gaining a better understanding of the actual cause of low back pain conditions, doctors and people suffering from these conditions can significantly improve their outcomes. I know this is possible from our own experience.

I want to take this opportunity to publicly thank Dr. Natalie and Dr. Lee for writing this book with me. Without their expertise and diverse training, this book would have never become a reality.

Below are the ten core principles that we have developed based on our findings.

TEN CORE PRINCIPLES

1. The cushions between the spinal bones are damaged in almost all back pain conditions.

In more detail: almost all chronic low back pain conditions involve, at some level, the intervertebral disc (which cushion adjacent vertebrae and act as spinal shock absorbers). Regardless of where the pain is being generated from—the disc, the nerves, the muscles or fascia surrounding the muscles— the disc is usually involved.

2. When the spine becomes unstable it will lead to chronic low back pain. An unstable spine is mechanically imbalanced.

In more detail: mechanical imbalance of the spine causes uneven pressure and shearing stresses to the intervertebral discs and surrounding spinal structures. These unbalanced forces, over time, damage the disc, causing excessive wear and stress to the disc and spinal structures (disc decay). This, in turn, leads to herniations, sciatica, stenosis, inflammation, and scar-tissue adhesions. Discs do not deteriorate with age; they deteriorate because of mechanical imbalances of the spine.

3. A group of highly specialized muscles are in charge of stabilizing the spine.

In more detail: in the past it was believed that ligaments (the leather strappings that hold bones together) were responsible for stabilizing the spine. We now know that the deep spinal muscles (deep multifidi, rotatores, and intertransversarii) are responsible for stability and coordinated movement of the spine. When these muscles become underactive or fire in an uncoordinated fashion, spinal decay will eventually follow.

4. Spinal balance and stability is not under our direct control.

In more detail: The central nervous system, or more specifically the autonomic control centers of the brain, directs and coordinates the firing patterns of the deep spinal-stabilizer muscles. This occurs without conscious effort just like our heart rate, digestion and blood pressure.

5. An unbalanced nervous system will always destabilize the spine.

In more detail: If the autonomic control centers of the brain become unbalanced (dysautonomia), mechanical imbalance of the spine (dyskinematics) will be one of the many consequences. We term the process of dysautonomia leading to dyskinematics as Neuromechanical Imbalance.

6. To successfully treat low back pain, the nervous system must be balanced as well as the deep spinal muscles.

In more detail: Successful treatment of any chronic low back condition requires a two-step approach. First, heal the damaged structures as much as is possible (the discs, vertebrae, muscles, fascia); second, restore neuromechanical balance to the spine. In order to properly implement the two-part approach, we must be able to measure and quantify the Neuromechanical Imbalance. New technology has now made accurate assessment of Neuromechanical Imbalances possible.

7. An unbalanced spine will always lead to an unbalanced nervous system, and an unbalanced nervous system will always lead to an unbalanced spine.

In more detail: Spinal decay is a symptom of a larger problem. It is the canary in the mine shaft signaling that the deep structures in the brain are not operating in a coordinated, healthy, fashion. Direct or repetitive trauma to the spine will lead to mechanical imbalances, which in turn, will lead to imbalances in the nervous system (proprioceptive deficits). This will lead to a host of other health problems, not just back pain. On the other hand, an unbalanced nervous system will over time lead to an unbalanced spine. An unbalanced spine is an unbalanced brain, and an unbalanced brain is an unbalanced spine.

8. Chronic stress is the number one cause of nervous system imbalance.

In more detail: Chronic stress leads to dysautonomia (unbalanced autonomic function). Stress physiologists call this process allostatic load. The devastating effects of allostatic load to our overall health and well-being, not only our spine, have been well documented in the recent scientific literature. Chronic stress is usually associated with psychological stress; this is a common misconception. Psychological stress is only the tip of the iceberg and accounts for only a small part of the total stress load. This is why the often-prescribed meditation and deep-breathing techniques, although somewhat effective, do not go far enough in reducing the chronic stress load.

9. An unbalanced nervous system (created from chronic stress) is the primary cause of at least 75 percent of all chronic diseases *(Sapolsky 2004, 6; Chestnut 2005, 54-55; McEwen et al. 2012; Karlamangla et al. 2002, 696-710 and more.)*

In more detail: Dysautonomia due to chronic stress is linked to most chronic and autoimmune diseases including cognitive decline (dementia), arthritis, spinal decay, diabetes, and cardiovascular disease to name a few. The damage caused from chronic stress—such as spinal decay, diabetes, etc.—itself becomes an internal stressor that further contributes to the overall chronic stress load. This creates a self-perpetuating, vicious cycle we term the chronic stress cycle. This destructive cycle cements a continuing stress response into our physiology.

10. You cannot escape from chronic stress in modern society, but you can dramatically reduce its effects.

In more detail: We live in a very different world than our great grandparents' world. Even though we are living longer due to modern medicine's advances in treating acute infections and trauma and improved hygiene practices, chronic disease (due to the chronic stress cycle) is on the rise (Gruenewald 2006; Karatsoreos, McEwen 2011; Karlamangla et al 2002; Singer, Ryff, Seeman 2004; Sterling 2004). We are living longer, but we are becoming increasingly sicker and losing our vitality and vigor for life at a much earlier age than we should (Crimmins and Beltrán-Sánchez 2010). Treating and managing our Neuromechanical Imbalances allows us a window into our nervous system. Addressing these imbalances gives us a more direct and effective way to balance the autonomic centers and break the chronic stress cycle. As you will soon discover, the health benefits of this process go well beyond just relieving low back pain.

This book is divided into three parts. Part one describes how Neuromechanical Imbalance causes spinal decay, as well as how to effectively treat these imbalances and restore spinal health. Part two explores how chronic stress, and more specifically the chronic stress cycle, causes Neuromechanical Imbalance. This section also demonstrates how the chronic stress cycle is the underlying cause of most chronic diseases. The last section, part three, gives you tools and strategies to reduce the chronic stress in your life.

In an effort to be thorough, this book covers a lot of territory. For a quick overview of how Neuromechanical Imbalance is evaluated and treated, we recommend reading chapter 1, and then skipping to chapter 11.

If you want a better understanding of how chronic stress causes low back pain, as well as most other chronic diseases, read part two.

For health-care providers working with low back pain, we would recommend reading through the book in a linear fashion and reviewing the research references that we have provided.

Part three is designed to be a stand-alone section that can be used as a home resource guide. You can pick and choose different strategies that fit your lifestyle and begin to take control of the chronic stressors in your life.

God Bless,

Russ Horine
August 10, 2014

P.S.
Janet, the nurse, made a full and complete recovery. She no longer experiences back pain or takes any medication. Not only is she back to 100 percent in tennis, cycling and hiking, when she comes in for her periodic check-ups she gets a kick out of sharing photos and stories of her new hobby… whitewater rafting!

PART I

NEUROMECHANICAL BALANCE AND SPINAL HEALTH

CHAPTER 1

BACK PAIN – THE COST

Do you, or somebody you know, suffer from back pain? Considering you're holding this book right now, we're pretty sure that you do. An astounding 85 percent of the US population suffers from back pain at some point in their lives *(Vallfors 1985; Eskay-Auerbach 2005; AANS 2011)*. In fact back problems are the second most common reason why people visit their doctor's office each day.

HERE ARE A FEW FACTS YOU SHOULD KNOW.

- Sixty-seven percent of people with first-time back pain will end up with chronic back pain problems *(Itz, et al 2013, 5–15)*.
- Back pain is *rarely* due to a bone or muscle problem *(Borkan and Van Tulder, et al. 2002, 128–132)*.
- The cause of back pain often does not show up on X-ray or MRI *(Frymoyer 1988, 291–300), (Mooney 1987, 754–59; Jensen et al. 1994, 69–73)*.
- Degeneration of the spine is *not* linked with old age. Spinal decay can occur at *any* age *(Twomey and Taylor*

1985, 496–499; Shao and Rompe and Schiltenwolf 2002, 263–8).

- There have been a growing number of children found with degenerative changes within the spine *(Alyas and Turner and Connell 2007, 836–41), (Rajeswaran et al. 2014, 925–32), (Waris et al. 2007, 681–4).*

With such a great percentage of our country, alone, suffering from the various forms of back pain, it's amazing the media has not talked about it as much as anti-aging or celebrity gossip. Without NBC news, *The View*, or Dr. Oz programs talking about the prevention, plausible causes, or treatment options, how is one supposed to know how to defeat this pain in the back?

Luckily, you have an array of pain-killers that can mask the problem since conventional medicine continues to mistakenly advocate the use of antidepressants, pain-killers, or both for chronic back pain *(Malanga and Wolf 2008, 173–84).* With "cures" like this, it is no wonder why there is an epidemic of prescription drug abuse.

Maybe you fall into the category of people who have suffered far too long, lost hope, and are now considering surgery as an option. Did you know that studies have confirmed that approximately *40 percent* of spinal surgeries are unnecessary? Maybe that is a clue as to why such a large percentage of spinal surgeries have failed. A recent review that was conducted by two doctors out of Johns Hopkins University details their concern for this growing number of failures—what they call "failed back surgery syndrome." Their review states that the growing number of low back surgeries being performed is expected to also have the same disappointing results *(Hussain and Erdek 2014, 64–78).* In fact unsuccessful back surgeries are so common that "failed back surgery syndrome" has become a diagnosis in and of itself and has its own insurance code!

What may seem like an obvious option for eliminating pain is now often shown to be unnecessary and more harmful than beneficial to one's health. And this information is coming from the very surgeons who are performing these surgeries.*

At the risk of sounding cynical, spinal surgeries have become a huge and much-needed revenue source for hospitals and surgeons. In 2013 alone over 3.5 billion dollars was spent on just one type of spinal surgery (spinal fusions). It just so happens that this is the same surgery that has one of the highest complication rates and poorest long-term outcomes. Yet surprisingly (and unfortunately) it has the highest insurance payouts for surgeons and hospitals *(PEPPER 2013)*.

Few people know what options are available and how to not become another back-pain statistic. More importantly, even fewer know why the pain occurs in the first place, let alone what to do about it.

Even when people try to be proactive in searching for better options, they are often led to the same ineffective treatment strategies. For instance, if you type *back pain* into your computer's search engine, the following treatment options will commonly show up: drugs, spinal injections, surgeries, lotions and potions, back rubs, and miraculous exercises.

Don't misunderstand; there are highly effective treatment options available. We know this from experience (and see it every day in our office). However, these treatment strategies are not widely known. It's no wonder that people who suffer

---

* There are some circumstances where the disc is so far damaged that nonsurgical recovery is not an option. In cases such as this, microsurgery should be explored as a first option.

from chronic back pain experience so much confusion, bad information, frustration, and misery.

THE REAL COST OF BACK PAIN

Back pain is not simply a pain that is located in your back; it affects all other aspects of your life. Back pain, for many, has created a loss of income by compromising their ability to work or causing them to be passed up for promotions because of too many sick days. If you experience chronic back pain, you may no longer be able to engage in recreational activities such as fishing, golfing, traveling, or bowling. Perhaps playing with your kids or grandkids has become more of a burden than a pleasure because you suffer the consequences after every family event. Or maybe your relationship with your spouse has been compromised because he or she simply cannot help you feel better (in spite of best efforts), is becoming worn out from having to do twice the work in the home, and is tired of hearing you complain. Simple tasks such as taking out the garbage, walking the dog, gardening, and running errands are no longer simple and require careful planning to avoid or reduce pain. And it gets worse…

You and 85 percent of the rest of the population have lost vitality, energy, and the zest for life because of constant pain. You may have been placed on antidepressants (and heavy pain medications) because you're now depressed from not being able to function and enjoy life's pleasures as you once did. You not only suffer emotionally and physically but also mentally. In fact there have been numerous studies linking chronic pain with cognitive decline (decreased memory, focus, and attention) *(Hart and Wade and Martelli; Gibbons 2003, 116-226).*

We understand why your back pain is more than just an inconvenience and discomfort. It affects *all* aspects of life.

COMMON TYPES OF BACK PAIN

Back pain can present with different types of pain patterns. The most common include:

- Disc pain—Pain that may or may not hurt in the center of your low back, but can also cause pain in the buttocks and hip
- Sciatica—The well-known pattern of shooting pain or numbness down the back or side of your leg that can reach as far as the big toe
- Central stenosis—Dull, achy pain that wraps around the front of the thighs and/or into the groin and down to the knee
- Facet pain—Sharp pain that occurs in the center of the low back and may travel into the hip(s)
- Sacroiliac pain—Pain that, like central stenosis, can present around the groin but is also localized in the sacroiliac joint affected and possibly into the buttock
- Fascial adhesions—Pain from adhesions is dependent on the locations of the adhesions and can travel anywhere throughout the back.

THE REAL PROBLEM

All of these conditions are intimately related to the intervertebral disc—the cushions between your spinal bones. When the disc becomes stressed and inflamed, it can lead to all of the back pain varieties described above. And it's important to note that this will always occur before it will show up on an MRI or X-ray. Once the disc is damaged, it will continue to progress eventually leading to the various forms of spinal decay that are included in the title of this book. In other words any successful treatment plan must include healing the disc.

It may surprise you to know that recent research has shown that all of these back pain conditions are ultimately being caused by an imbalanced nervous system. When the nervous system becomes imbalanced, the spine, which it controls, becomes imbalanced. An imbalanced spine creates friction, inflammation, and damage to the disc leading to the aforementioned back pain varieties. Together, an imbalanced spine and nervous system is called a *Neuromechanical Imbalance.*

Once again, any successful treatment plan must resolve the Neuromechanical Imbalance in addition to restoring the disc. If your disc is addressed without correcting the Neuromechanical Imbalance, then your back pain will eventually return. The good news is, if caught in its early stages, simply correcting the Neuromechanical Imbalance alone can restore the disc.

The bad news is if the Neuromechanical Imbalance is allowed to persist, the nervous system no longer has the ability to control all of the unconscious, automatic functions of the body in a highly fine-tuned manner as it once did. This is referred to as *dysautonomia* and has serious, far-reaching health consequences that can destroy your quality of life in more ways than your back-pain symptoms alone.

In this book you'll learn that your back pain, sciatica, herniations, stenosis, and so on are caused by something much greater. We will also discuss the recent research findings that relate the Neuromechanical Imbalance to chronic diseases such as diabetes, heart disease, cognitive decline, depression, loss of energy, and more.

WHY HAVEN'T YOU HEARD ABOUT NEUROMECHANICAL IMBALANCE?

You haven't heard of it because we *created* the term. Let us explain...

The fact is that researchers in different fields of study have been talking about this concept for years. The problem is that the researchers have not explored outside their professional sandbox. The research world tends to be confined to chosen specialties. For example, those in the field of kinesiology focus all of their time and energy in the world of kinesiology. Likewise, researchers in the field of neuroscience spend their life in the "box" of neuroscience. Because of this, there is little cross talk or cross research among different specialties.

To make matters worse, each specialty has its own unique language that is used to describe the same or similar processes. This further discourages the free flow of information between different specialties.

In order to improve our clinical outcomes, we were forced to overcome this trap of specialization and look outside our sandbox. We explored the research of other specialties, which allowed us to connect the dots.

After connecting the dots, we were taken aback with what we had found.

While some specialties focused more on the *neuro* part, others focused on the *mechanical* part. This division among fields of study led to many different terms for the brain-spine connection such as: vertebral subluxation complex, dyskinematics, allostatic load, hemisphericity, cortical desynchronization, proprioceptive deficit, and dysautonomia.

These different fields of study were exploring the concepts of what we have coined, for simplicity and clarity, *Neuromechanical Imbalance.*

We used research from stress physiology, neuroscience, kinesiology, functional neurology, chiropractic, and manual medicine to create the most effective approach to treating low back pain that we have seen in over thirty years of clinical experience.

We have also discovered that by addressing the neuro part of Neuromechanical Imbalance, we have been able to consistently improve a low-back-pain sufferer's energy, vitality, health, and quality of life in ways that were even surprising to us.

THE LAYOUT OF THIS BOOK

We've done our best to make this book nontechnical; however there is an extensive amount of material that we must include for the sake of thoroughness. The following is a brief overview of the different sections of the book.

PASSIVE AND ACTIVE SYSTEMS

Part one of this book provides a basic overview of spinal anatomy and introduces you to the passive and active systems of the back. The passive system includes the ligaments, joints, discs, and fascia, while the active system encompasses the nervous system and the muscles it controls. We refer to the active system as the *neuromechanical system.*

In low back conditions, pain typically arises from the passive system. And you will learn that the disc, a passive structure, is nearly always involved. You will also learn that damage to the passive structures almost always develops as a direct result of imbalance of the active system—the neuromechanical system.

The past mistake was to direct treatment to the passive system for two reasons. One, the pain in the back came from the passive system; therefore, the squeaky wheel got the grease. And two, the traditional methods used to evaluate low back pain relied on X-rays, MRIs, and simple orthopedic tests to find the problem. The mistake here is that these evaluations only look at the passive system—which is a downstream consequence of the upstream problem. These tests give no information about the neuromechanical system, which led to the damaged passive system in the first place.

This mistake is understandable because Neuromechanical Imbalance was not well understood, and it was difficult to measure in the clinical setting.

Heart rate variability, surface EMGs, tissue perfusion, skin conductance, and functional neurological tests—some of the tools that can measure Neuromechanical Imbalance—were not widely available until recently. So it is completely understandable why the Neuromechanical Imbalance has been ignored for so long.

With the emergence of new technology and a better understanding of the nervous system, we can now accurately measure the neuromechanical system using more precise tools and tests.

A doctor cannot effectively treat a condition that can't be measured. This exciting new technology has been a breakthrough for the clinicians in the field. Now, for the first time ever, the neuromechanical system can be effectively evaluated and restored.

Our Two-Part Approach to
Treating Low Back Pain

Before the end of part one, we dedicate an entire chapter to the cause of almost all back-pain issues—the Neuromechanical Imbalance. We provide diagrams for ease of understanding and explain how Neuromechanical Imbalances are the basis of your back pain.

In the last chapter of part one, we outline our two-part approach to treating low back pain. This approach is dedicated to taking care of both the active and passive systems. We address the damage to the disc and other structures with the latest technology and therapies including super-pulsed cold laser; targeted, high-speed-pressure wave therapy; manual and tool-assisted flexion-distraction therapies; myofascial-release techniques; and spinal mobilizations. Depending on the severity of the disc damage, computer-controlled spinal-decompression therapy may be an important adjunct to healing the disc damage.

With the new tools available to us for evaluating the neuromechanical system, the clinician can now look at all the different treatments available and determine what actually works. In our office we have spent the last four years developing a collection of therapies that have proven themselves to be effective through objective testing and better clinical outcomes. Because neuromechanical integration is a mouthful, we casually refer to them as *balancing therapies*.

The conclusion of this chapter sets a foundation for part two, which reveals the cause of Neuromechanical Imbalance—*chronic stress*. It will also illuminate the unexpected connection between low back pain and chronic disease.

Fasten your seat belt because this gets interesting.

How Chronic Stress Leads to Chronic Disease

In part two we demonstrate the well-established connection between chronic stress and disease. In fact, authorities in the field now recognize that a majority of all chronic diseases—including cardiovascular disease, diabetes, degenerative joint disease, arthritis, and mental decline, among others—are caused from chronic stress *(Sapolsky 2004, 6; Chestnut 2005, 54-55; McEwen et al. 2012; Karlamangla et al. 2002, 696-710 and more)*. Chronic stress wreaks havoc by throwing the autonomic nervous system off balance.

The autonomic nervous system is responsible for all of the automatic, unconscious functions of the body including hormone regulation, digestion, body temperature, blood pressure, and so on.

Therefore, when chronic stress triggers *autonomic imbalance* (also called *allostatic load* in research), it will eventually lead to some type of chronic disease including *mechanical imbalances*. The process of autonomic imbalance creating mechanical imbalance is the more precise definition of *Neuromechanical Imbalance*.

The amazing benefit of measuring and treating the autonomic imbalance allows us to have a significant impact on a person's overall health, much greater than treating back pain alone.

Things You Can Do at Home to Decrease the Stress Response

Part three is a jammed-pack protocol full of tools and strategies that you can use right now at home to decrease your autonomic imbalance and chronic stressors. We call this the DICE protocol, and it addresses four primary factors that have been shown to consistently lower chronic stress.

We lay out, in detail, how to improve sleep, posture, breathing, and diet. *Deep sleep* is essential for healing and restoration. *Inline posture* is necessary for balanced brain function. *Complete breathing* provides the proper amount of oxygen necessary for optimum brain function. *Energy diet* is a simple and easy eating strategy that encourages healing and supplies clean fuel to your energy-starved cells.

At the end of part three, we will cover easy, home exercises that are an integral part of our treatment program. These exercises are not included in the DICE protocol because getting out of acute pain is necessary before a successful exercise program can be implemented. Exercising in pain has been shown to strengthen pain pathways, which can reinforce chronic pain and lead to chronic pain syndromes. (The pain remains even when the problem is removed.)

At the end of the book, we include a resource section on products and services we have found valuable for decreasing environmental stressors.

Now that you have a clear overview of where we are going, let's get started with learning some basic anatomy. We promise this won't be painful. We have only provided the essential pieces necessary to provide you with a basic understanding of your incredible spine.

Now let's get started.

CHAPTER 2

HOW OUR SPINE WORKS

KEY POINTS

- The spine is designed to provide a strong, yet mobile, foundation to the body to allow you to walk upright. It also anchors the arms and legs to the body.
- You have twenty-four movable bones in your spine called vertebrae. The ones in your low back are called *lumbar vertebrae*. In your neck they are called *cervical vertebrae*, and in your midback they are called *thoracic vertebrae*.
- Between each vertebra you have a sponge-like *disc* that acts like a shock absorber and allows the vertebrae to move without touching each other.
- Ligaments and muscles hold bones together. The muscles are responsible for movement and stability of your joints, whereas the ligaments protect against excessive motion such as overextension.
- Fascia is the tissue between all of the other tissues like bone, muscles, and ligaments that wraps them all together so everything stays in its proper place.

- Your pelvis is made up of three major bones with three joints to relieve pressure and allow for a little extra give.
- The spinal cord, which is an extension of the brain, is located inside the hollow part of the spine for protection.
- Nerves from the spinal cord exit the vertebrae through gaps between the vertebrae called intervertebral foramen.
- The brain is the master controller of the entire body, and it sends and receives messages to the muscles, organs, and glands via the spinal cord and nerves.

Now we need to provide you with a very brief introduction to the anatomy of spine and its counterparts. This introduction will allow you to become familiar with terms and concepts that will be addressed in a much more digestible fashion later. We don't intend for you to master anatomy; however, it's helpful to have some reference to the basics in order to get a clear picture of how your spine works. You can skip this section if you like, but be sure to use it as a reference if you come across unclear concepts later.

Are you ready? Here we go.

The human spine defies gravity like a modern-day skyscraper. Think about the ingenuity that went into constructing the Empire State Building. How can a building like that maintain its structure against gravity, rain, wind, or horrific snowstorms? Architects understood the concepts of *structural support* within this building. Structural support is what our spine provides for our bodies on a day-to-day basis. It actually differentiates us in the animal kingdom by way of our vertical bipedalism (upright walking with two feet). We are the only species that is able to stand upright while bending, twisting, or performing any of our activities throughout the day.

The spinal column consists of intervertebral discs (discs for short) and twenty-four movable vertebrae in the neck, middle back, and low back. There are seven vertebrae that make up the neck known as the cervicals, twelve for the midback known as the thoracics, and five in the low back called the lumbar spine. The rest include five fused vertebrae that form the sacrum and four that are fused to create the coccyx (tail bone).

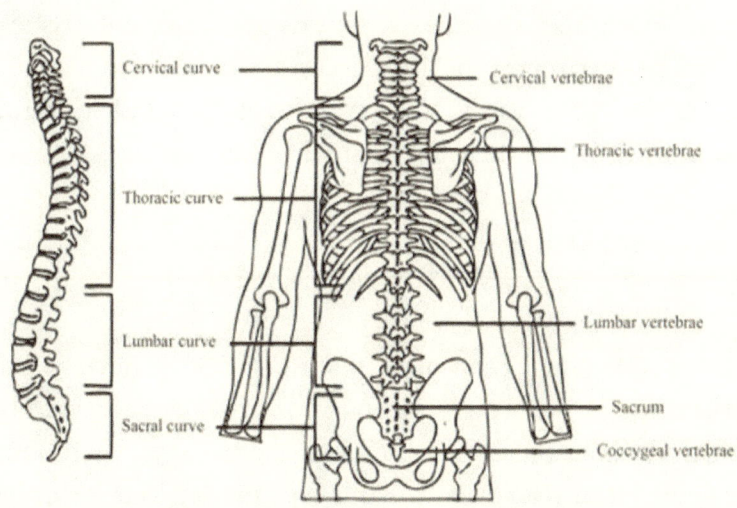

Notice the triangular shaped bone in between the hip bones in the picture above? That is the sacrum. The pointed section below that is the coccyx. Your spine (aka spinal column) reaches from the bottom tip of the coccyx to the very top vertebrae (atlas).

Most spinal columns consist of twenty-four total vertebrae, but some people have an extra or a missing vertebra. The mid twelve vertebrae make up your midback and provide attachment sites for the ribs that protect your vital organs. At the sacrum the ilia (hip bones) are connected on either side creating the pelvis. The pelvis is like a basin that holds other vital structures—such as the reproductive organs and bladder—in addition to providing a place for the thigh bone (femur) to attach. Take another look at the previous picture.

The spine forms the connection of the upper and lower portions of your body. In other words the arms and legs both anchor to the spine, which in turn connects them both. This is an important concept that we will later explore to understand how an injury in the lower half of the body can eventually affect the upper half and vice versa.

The spine also provides locations for different tissues to attach. These special types of tissues are called connective tissues, and they provide the body with stability and movement. These include discs, muscles, ligaments, and fascia.

What Is the Disc?

If there is one part of the spine that most people have heard of, it is the intervertebral discs, the cushions between the vertebrae. You have twenty-three discs in total, one between each bone in your spine from your head to your sacrum. In your lower back, these five little shock-absorbing cushions add about two inches to the lumbar spine. Have you ever wondered why some people lose height with age? Well, it's due to the breakdown of these discs, mostly in the low back and lower neck. Since the low back is at the bottom of the totem pole, the discs here are thicker and stronger in order to hold up the extra weight of our torso. It makes sense that most disc problems occur at the bottom of the spine. In fact 96.7 percent of all spinal surgeries are attempts to repair damage in the bottom two discs alone *(Wheeler 2013)*!

Normal Vertebral Segment
(Front View)

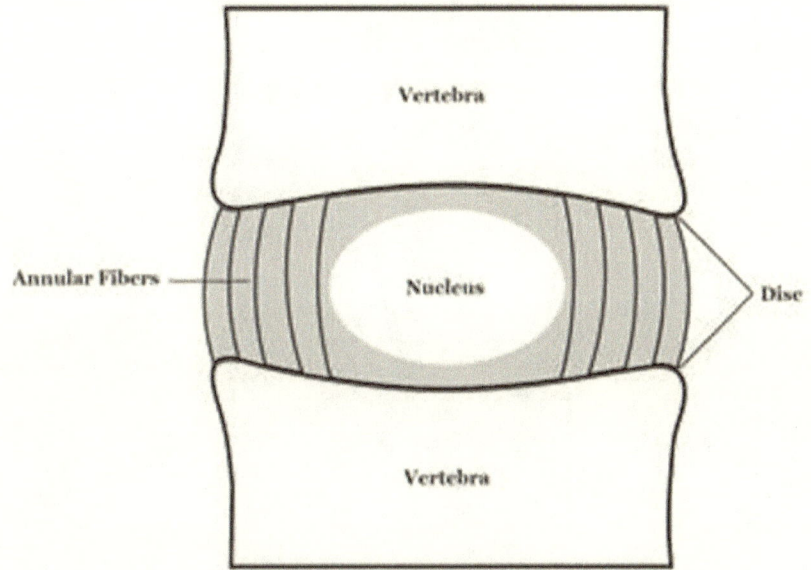

Vertebra

Annular Fibers

Nucleus

Disc

Vertebra

TENDONS AND MUSCLES

There are one hundred forty-four muscles in the entire body, and each one has two tendons. Tendons are the anchors that attach a muscle to a bone. Generally speaking, when a muscle contracts, it shortens, moving the bone closer to another bone. When it lengthens it does the opposite.

Most muscles and tendons are responsible for movement; however, some are specifically designed for stability. When it comes to muscles in the spine, they are layered like a stack of pancakes. Specialized stability muscles are located at the bottom of the stack, closest to the spine. This gives them a strategic advantage in creating stability. The spinal muscles further away from the spine have more leverage (just like grabbing a crowbar at the end gives you more leverage) and are responsible for creating movement.

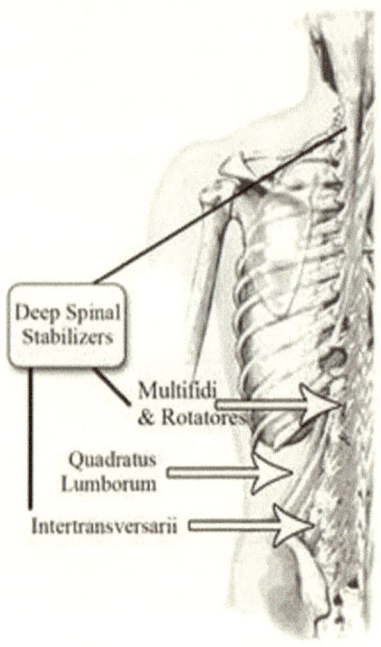

It is also helpful to understand that each of these stability muscles are very small, and in addition to providing stability, they act as a sensor for the brain, telling the brain how the spine is moving. These muscles are important, and we will revisit them in future chapters.

LIGAMENTS AND JOINTS

Ligaments are the connective tissues that connect a bone to another bone—just like tape is used to connect two flaps of a cardboard box. There are hundreds of ligaments located throughout the body that connect two bones together to create a *joint*. This is also known as an articulation. Every joint in the body is taped together by ligaments and reinforced by the muscles. Together, ligaments and muscles are responsible for keeping joints like your knees, elbows, and spinal vertebrae held together.

FASCIA

This is the plastic wrap and glue that holds *everything* together. For years, anatomists and doctors alike considered fascia to be an unimportant tissue that served no major purpose. It wasn't until recently that fascia was rediscovered.

We now know that fascia has nerves; it moves, and it is a critical component of the overall integrity of the body. In fact new anatomists have shown that the body is connected via the fascia from your head to your toes. The rediscovery of fascia has also reminded us that the body is one big connected piece. Breaking it down into smaller components is simply a convenience of study.

Now that we have talked about some of the connective tissues, let's revisit the bony aspects of the spine that are critical to understanding your low back pain.

CERVICAL, THORACIC, AND LUMBAR VERTEBRAE

The following sections make up the majority of the spine: cervical, thoracic, and lumbar vertebrae. Despite their separate locations throughout the spine, every vertebra is connected by way of the large muscles, ligaments, discs, and fascia surrounding them. Because of this connection, a disruption in the lower spine can affect areas in the upper spine due to the dynamic relationship they share. In fact since the arms and legs are anchored to the spine via fascia, muscles, and ligaments, disruption of the spine can cause injuries and dysfunction in the arms or legs.

Let's take a deeper look at the low back.

There are five vertebrae in the low back that make up the lumbar spine. The lumbar vertebrae are located between the ribs and sacrum as illustrated in the picture below.

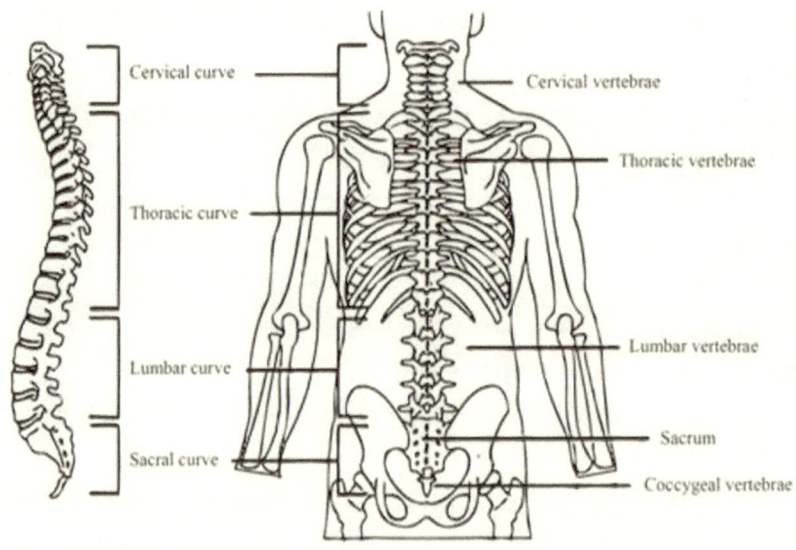

As you can see, the lumbar vertebrae are larger than the rest. This is because they are the vertebrae bearing the most weight within the spine (aside from the sacrum), and they are designed to most efficiently disperse the weight from gravity and the body. You can compare this concept to a pyramid; the bottom must be larger in order to form a strong foundation to handle the weight of all the stones above it. In the spine, weight transfer continues its way through the lumbar vertebrae and into the top of the sacrum, eventually being transferred into the hips. As we mentioned earlier, the bottom lumbar vertebrae are most susceptible to injury and pain.

The lumbar spine provides a direct connection to the lower limb by way of the iliopsoas muscle. This muscle is responsible for bringing the thigh toward the hip. Again this emphasizes how important the role of the spine is in providing stability to the lower (and upper) limbs. So the lumbar spine must be really strong to tolerate holding up the weight of the torso as well as to act as an anchor to the legs.

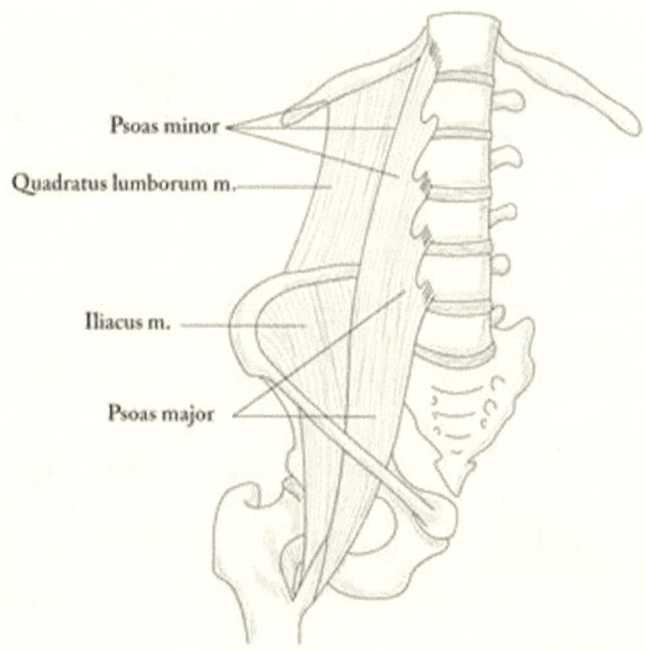

Psoas minor
Quadratus lumborum m.
Iliacus m.
Psoas major

PELVIS, PUBIC SYMPHYSIS, AND SACROILIAC JOINTS

The pelvis, which is created by the hip bones and sacrum, attaches the lower limbs to the rest of the body. The two hip bones are joined to the sacrum in the back to form the sacroiliac joint, whereas the front connection forms the pubic symphysis.

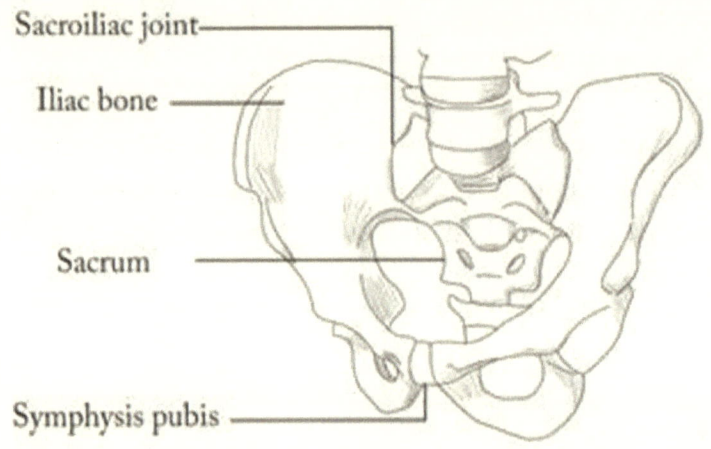

Sacroiliac joint

Iliac bone

Sacrum

Symphysis pubis

The top of the hip bone (iliac crest) and pubic symphysis serve as attachment sites for the abdominal wall muscles known as the obliques, transversus abdominis, and the rectus abdominis. These front muscles, in addition to others in the back, contribute to core stability and will be discussed thoroughly in upcoming chapters.

The sacroiliac joints and pubic symphysis move slightly to relieve pressure in the pelvis, which prevents it from breaking from too much stress. This is the same principle used for the construction of a bridge that is engineered with joints that allow for more flexibility without breaking.

The back of the hip bone provides attachments for your gluteal or buttock muscles that help you tuck your hips while standing upright or performing a back kick in martial arts. These direct muscle attachments, with their overlying fascia, can be associated with low back pain.

FACET JOINTS

These joints are positioned in the back of the spine and are formed by the lower part of the top vertebra and the upper portion of the vertebra below

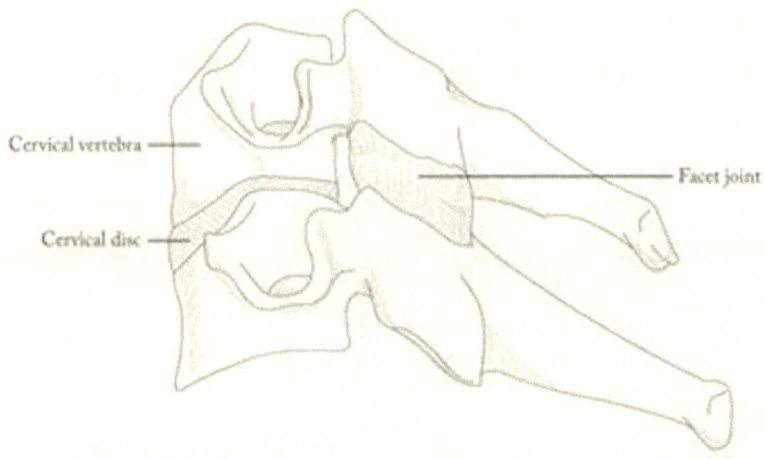

Just like most joints, these should have a nice space in between them. They are slightly load bearing in the spine, meaning that they help to transfer some body weight and assist the intervertebral discs. When there is no space, problems develop that we will discuss later.

There are two facet joints that are located on the back right and left portions of almost every vertebra. The key to these joints is that they are responsible for restriction and specificity of movement because of their varying orientations throughout the spine. In other words they limit how much your spine can bend and twist and act similarly to guide rails in a dresser drawer.

For example, the lumbar spine is made to resist excessive rotation and forward bending.

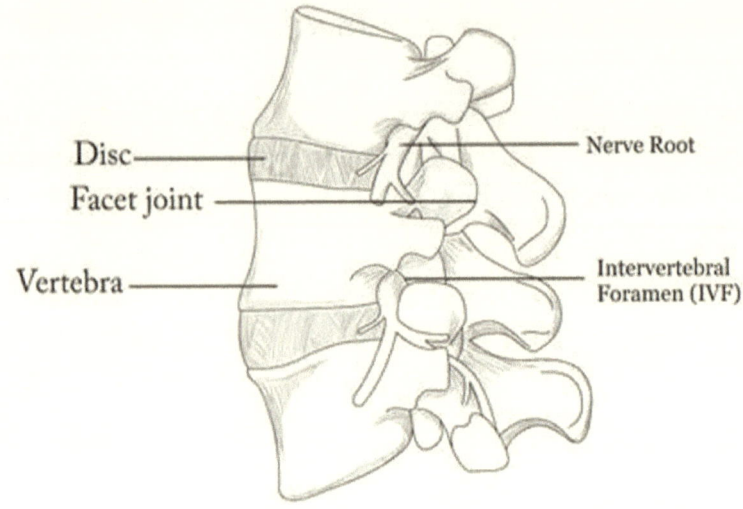

Disc —
Facet joint —
Vertebra —
Nerve Root
Intervertebral Foramen (IVF)

INTERVERTEBRAL FORAMEN (IVF)

These are right and left openings created by two adjoining vertebrae that are located between (inter-) each vertebra. They are the openings that allow the spinal nerves to exit at the level of the muscles for which they are responsible. This is why they are also referred to as neural (nerve) foramen.

Now all of this motion of the spine would not be made possible if it weren't for the power that turns the muscles on. This power is created from the brain-muscle connection, aka neuromuscular system. Let's do a very brief overview of this connection.

BRAIN, SPINAL CORD, AND NERVES

Just as the power station is responsible for providing power throughout the community, the brain is the organ responsible for sending power, in the form of electrical messages, throughout the body.

The brain talks to the muscles by way of the nerves exiting from particular levels of the spinal cord. Whenever a nerve exits the spinal cord, it will go to a specific destination. Therefore, doctors are able to track the level of nerve dysfunction depending on the muscles that are affected.

The electrical messages sent to the muscles not only turn them "on," but dictate how and when they will perform their jobs. Messages are constantly being sent throughout the entire body, in a matter of microseconds, so it can perform activities ranging from riding a bike to reading a book such as this.

The nerves are actually extensions from the spinal cord, which, in reality, is an extension of the brain. That being said, the messages from the brain must first travel through the spinal cord and then branch out to the appropriate nerve level.

Have a look at the picture below.

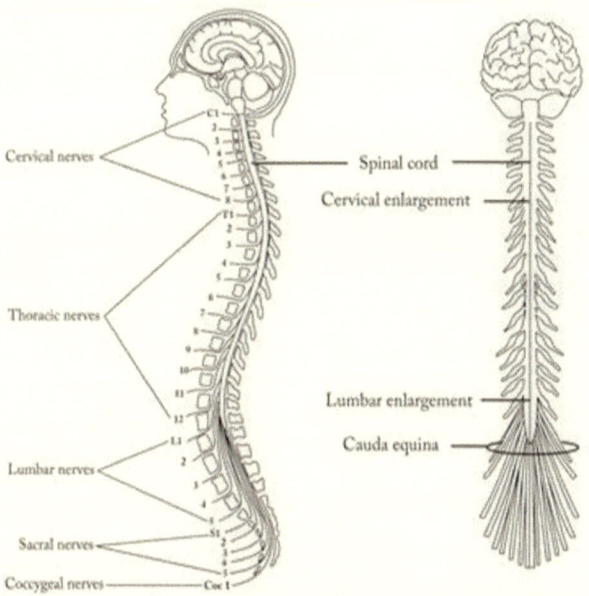

You may notice that nerves extend all that way down to your sacrum, but the spinal cord itself actually ends at your second lumbar vertebra. The nerves you see below that level are collectively called the *cauda equina*, which is Latin for "horse's tail." Regardless of the name, they are the nerves that transmit messages to other areas of the body, in this case the lower limbs.

The brain is encased and protected by the skull, whereas the spinal cord is protected by the spinal column. When we consider the importance of the nerves and spinal cord sending messages to and from the rest of the body, we can readily see that the spine is an important piece of real estate that works to protect the messages being sent, in addition to providing structural support. Therefore, it makes sense that maintaining the integrity of the spine is critical to protect these incoming and outgoing messages.

Now that we're through with our fast-track anatomy course, it's time to talk about the culprit of back pain.

CHAPTER 3

COMMON DIAGNOSES OF LOW BACK PAIN

KEY POINTS

- A disc herniation/bulging disc is when the inside of the disc (nucleus pulposus) pushes past the outer boundary of the disc causing the entire disc to bulge out.
- Disc herniations are caused by imbalanced pressure on the disc for long periods of time. They start as small tears and gradually get worse.
- Disc herniations cause pain that shoots into the buttock, thigh, and/or toes by pushing on sensitive nerves leaving the spine (nerve roots).
- Sciatica is the generalized term for pain that shoots down the buttock, thigh, or toes.
- Sciatica is caused by disc herniations and can usually be relieved by bending the body away from the bulge. This is why people with sciatica have to walk stooped over and crooked.

- Sitting tends to aggravate disc herniations because the disc is loaded with more weight than it can comfortably tolerate. Therefore, standing is usually more comfortable for people with sciatica.
- MRIs cannot accurately determine if there is a disc herniation.
- Spinal stenosis is the term used when a disc herniation pushes on the spinal cord, and it causes pain similar to sciatica. The pain is accompanied with a feeling of weakness in the upper thighs.
- Those with spinal stenosis feel better when they are leaning forward.
- Eighty-five percent of people with low back pain are diagnosed with *idiopathic low back pain*, which simply means, "I don't know why you have low back pain."
- If you are diagnosed with idiopathic low back pain or lumbalgia, seek out a different doctor.

In this chapter we will begin unraveling the mystery of how the low back fails.

Let's begin.

DISC HERNIATION

Disc herniation is a fairly common back complaint. You have probably heard of it or may possibly have it yourself. A herniated disc is sometimes referred to as a *slipped disc* or *bulging disc*, but the terms basically mean the same thing. A herniated disc happens when the jellylike nucleus pulposus squeezes out through tears in the annulus fibrosus (the tough outer ring that makes up one-third of the disc). The size of the tears, and how much fluid is in the disc, will determine the severity of the disc herniation.

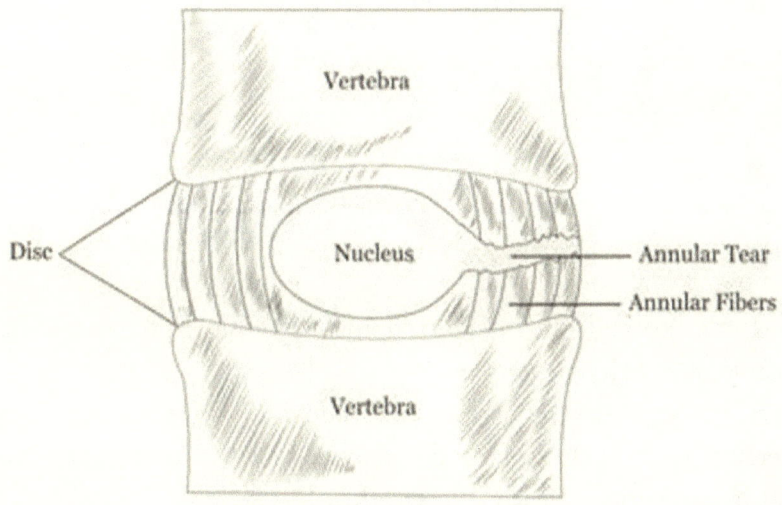

While it's beneficial to have more fluid in a disc, it can also lead to greater problems if there is a significant mechanical imbalance in the spine (where the vertebrae are not balanced evenly across the disc). The increased fluid in the center of the disc allows for greater pressure to push through the annular tears, and the disc is more likely to bulge out more severely. On the other hand, the more degenerated a disc becomes, the less jellylike fluid is in the nucleus pulposus, and therefore, there is less pressure exerted against the torn annular fibers. As a consequence a degenerated disc's ability to bulge out really far is limited. Think of the difference in difficulty in trying to pop a fully inflated balloon versus a just-shy of being fully deflated balloon. The inflated balloon is much easier to pop.

Side View of Vertebral Segments

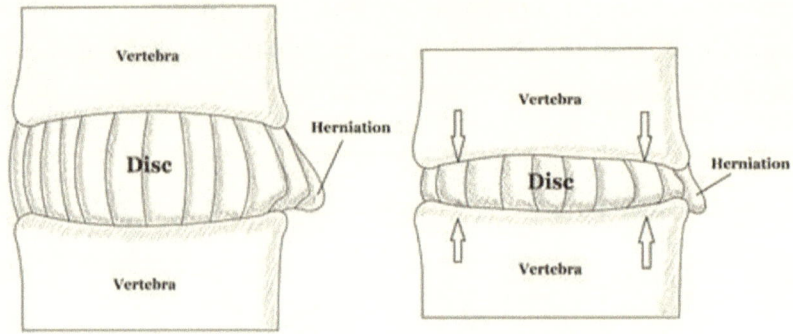

Disc Herniation without Degeneration   Disc Herniation with Degeneration
(Loss of disc height)

Let's expand on this balloon analogy a bit. Imagine the balloon is now full of jelly...

If you squeeze the balloon between your two flat hands symmetrically, the jelly is forced outward in all directions equally. But if you squeeze with one hand only, the jelly all squishes to the opposite side, putting excessive pressure on only one side of the balloon. The jelly wants to burst out, and if there is any weakness in the stressed area of the balloon, it will pop.

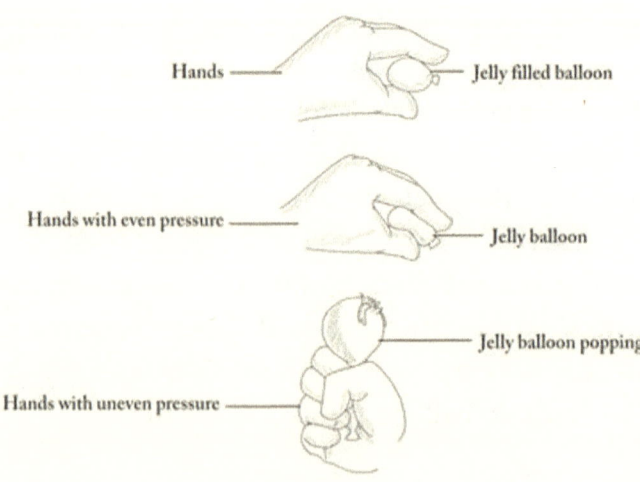

This is similar to how the disc behaves between the vertebral bodies. As we bend or lean, the jellylike fluid moves around in the disc allowing that movement to occur while maintaining a cushion for the spinal bones. If there is excessive pressure on one side of the disc, the nucleus pulposus will find relief from this pressure by shifting to the opposite side.

When uneven pressure is applied to the disc(s) for long periods of time (months or years), the inner part of the annulus begins to break down and tear. These microtears do not have enough time to repair, due to the constant stress of the mechanical imbalance pushing the jellylike fluid toward the small tears. At some point the tears become large enough that the pressure pushes the nucleus pulposus farther and farther into the tear causing the tears to expand.

Lumbar Disc Herniation

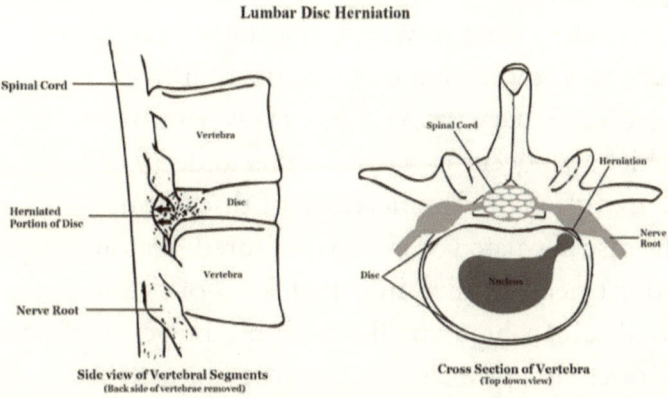

Spinal Cord

Vertebra

Disc

Herniated Portion of Disc

Vertebra

Nerve Root

Side view of Vertebral Segments
(Back side of vertebrae removed)

Spinal Cord

Herniation

Nerve Root

Disc

Nucleus

Cross Section of Vertebra
(Top down view)

As the jellylike fluid pushes through the tears, it creates a bulge in the outer ring of the disc, pushing outward from its normal position and into nearby structures such as nerve roots. The more the annulus tears, the bigger the bulge becomes. Its size is limited by how much fluid is in the disc (more fluid + tear = bigger herniation). It not only creates pain due to the tearing and inflammation in the disc but also due to the inflammation outside the disc.

In addition the classic presentation of disc herniation is shooting pain in the buttock, back of the thigh, and possibly down into the toes. This is caused by pressure from the bulging disc and the surrounding inflammation compressing or irritating the nerve roots that control the legs.

The nerve roots, which are the first nerve branches leaving the spinal cord, are highly susceptible to damage and irritation. Once these nerve roots exit the spine and join up with neighboring nerve roots to form a spinal nerve, they get bigger and have a strong protective sheath. This sheath is designed to be tough so that activities such as bending your knee or raising your leg don't damage the spinal nerve. However, before the nerve roots become a spinal nerve (and gain a protective sheath), they rely on the spinal bones (vertebrae) to protect them. This works well with a healthy disc; however, the unprotected nerve root is vulnerable to compression or inflammation from a damaged or bulging disc. A nerve root is especially sensitive to inflammation, which will occur as a disc begins to decay or herniates.

There are different classifications of disc herniations based on how the disc herniated or if it has ruptured. For our purposes here, we don't need to dive into that level of detail. Suffice it to say, the disc can be a small bulge, big bulge, or ruptured. Ruptured discs are problematic because the jellylike nucleus pulposus has literally broken out of the annulus and can leak out. As you can imagine, ruptured discs can be the most difficult forms to treat.

Sciatica

One of the most common ways people discover they have a herniated disc is when the bulge pushes into the big nerve of the leg. This creates a condition called sciatica, which is shooting pain down the buttock, thigh, and possibly into the foot. Sciatica derives its name from the nerve that goes into the leg called the sciatic nerve. This condition is extremely painful and can quite literally take you to the ground in agony. Nerves don't like to be squeezed, and as the disc herniates, it can compress the nerve roots that turn into the sciatic nerve, creating shooting leg pain in either one or both legs. There can be back pain associated with sciatica as well, but the lightning bolts firing into the leg often overshadow the back pain.

Sciatica can cause people to lean and contort their bodies in awkward ways to find relief. This is called antalgia. What's happening here is the person in pain is shifting pressures in the disc to decrease pressure on the sciatic nerve. The shifting basically serves to make the bulge smaller.

Left Sided, Lateral (away from center) Disc Herniation

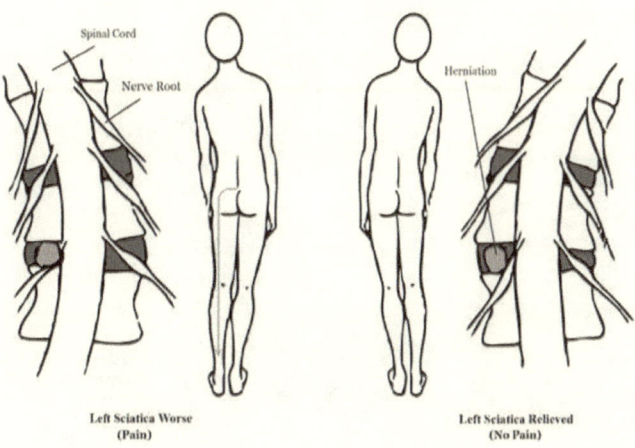

Left Sciatica Worse
(Pain)

Left Sciatica Relieved
(No Pain)

Most people with sciatic pain do not want to sit. Why is this? When you are standing, 60 percent of your upper-body weight is supported in the hips. When sitting, all the weight is supported in the lumbar spine and discs, so last thing you want to do is put all of your weight directly on the decayed discs. Standing relieves this excess pressure.

What seems strange is that oftentimes, on an MRI, the herniated disc doesn't even push on the sciatic nerve roots. Yet, the patient may still have the same shooting pain that is associated with sciatica. There are usually two major reasons for this. The first is that most MRIs are done with the person lying down, and the disc is no longer under the pressure that causes a bulge. So, unless the disc is extremely damaged, the bulge won't show up on MRI.* The second reason is a result of the inflammation we spoke of outside the disc. Just as inflammation inside the disc can cause severe pain in the low back, inflammation outside the disc can irritate the sciatic nerve roots causing shooting pain down the leg. When there is enough inflammation near the nerve roots, it will cause the same type of pain even if there isn't physical compression of the nerve.

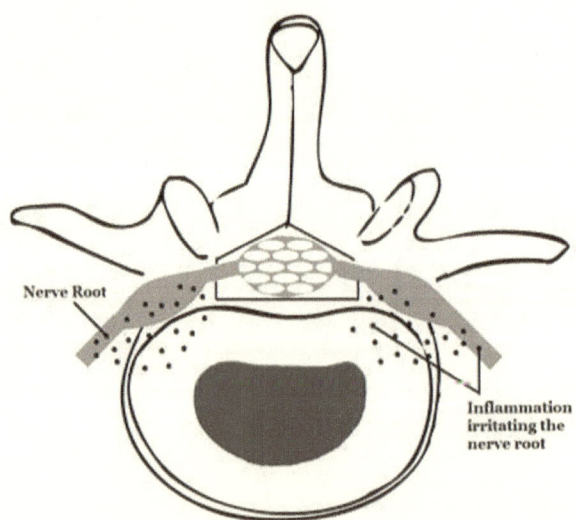

Cross Section of a Disc with Inflammation

---

* Radiologists who read the MRI must make their diagnoses based strictly on the images they see. Even if they understand that a bulge could be present if the patient were standing, they are not allowed to call it a herniation unless it shows up on the film.

SPINAL STENOSIS

Another common complication of a herniated disc is spinal stenosis. Spinal stenosis is the medical way of saying that the disc has bulged into the spinal canal. The spinal canal is where the spinal cord is housed. It seems obvious that we don't want any pressure on something as sensitive as the spinal cord, which is a major extension of the brain. The silver lining, if you want to stay positive, is that the spinal cord stops in the upper lumbar vertebrae.

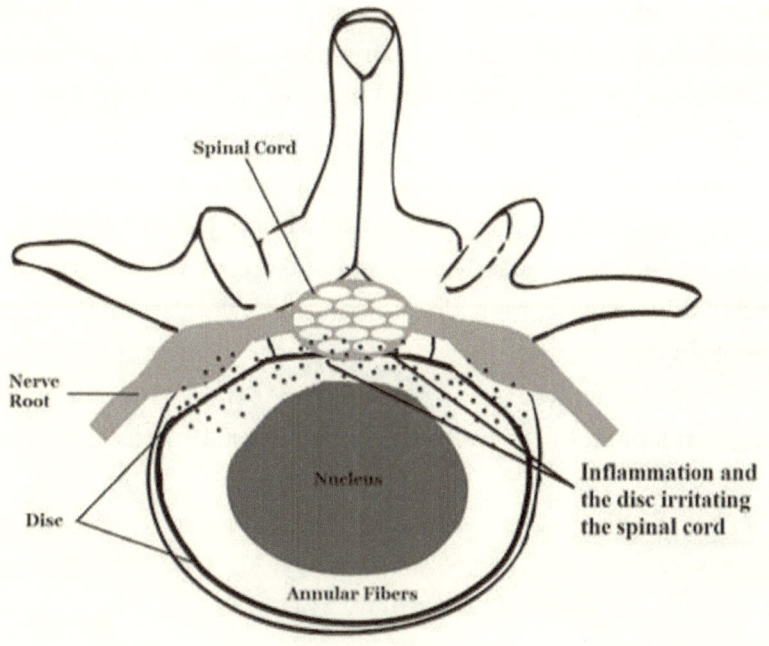

Spinal Stenosis

In the lower lumbar vertebrae (where almost all lumbar herniations occur), the spinal canal houses smaller branches of nerves that travel into the legs, so there is slightly more free space here than higher up in the spine. This allows for a little wiggle room before significant compression occurs. But this can still be an extremely dangerous condition if the herniation is large enough and directed back toward the spinal canal. Since these are the same nerves that control the bowel, bladder, and sexual function, in addition to the nerves in the legs, serious complications can arise if they are compressed.

Usually the major symptom of spinal stenosis is back pain with pain and that shoots into one or both legs, making it look very similar to sciatica—although the pain tends to be located more around the groin and front of the thighs. It usually feels best to lean forward, because this moves the nucleus pulposus away from the spinal cord and relieves some of the pressure. Furthermore, the pain is often accompanied by thigh weakness and aching, especially during standing and walking. But this type of pain is quickly relieved when sitting—which is the opposite of sciatica. As with sciatica there can be symptoms of spinal stenosis and pain due to inflammation around the disc. The pain can occur with or without physical compression of the disc. Either way, we can be certain that if there is sciatic pain or symptoms of stenosis, there will be inflammation in and around the disc.

IDIOPATHIC LOW BACK PAIN

Whenever you have a problem and doctors don't know why it is occurring, we don't officially say, "I don't know." Doctors are much more sophisticated than that; we say it in Greek.

Idiopathic literally translates to "one's own suffering," or a "disease of its own kind." It's all just a fancy way of saying that there is something wrong, but we don't know what is causing it.

Strangely, idiopathic is the most common diagnosis for low back pain in the medical world. If there isn't a blatantly obvious disc herniation, a tumor, fracture, inflammatory arthropathy, or significant degenerative disc disease (which most doctors wrongly consider to be a normal aging process), then medical doctors diagnose the condition as idiopathic low back pain, which sounds better than, "I don't know what's causing your back pain." Another official diagnosis they may use is lumbalgia.

Lumbalgia means *low back pain.*

How brilliant! You go to your doctor because you have low back pain, and he or she diagnoses you with low back pain, or back pain of unknown origin. Then you are sent home with some muscle relaxers and pain meds (both of which do absolutely nothing to fix the problem). This happens way too often. In fact research has shown that 85 percent of low back pain patients leave with a diagnosis of "I don't know" *(Binder and Nampiaparampil 2009, 15–24).*

As chiropractors specializing in low back pain, it's disappointing to us that anyone would be labeled as having idiopathic low back pain when there are only a handful of things that cause the pain. It's easy for us to understand the medical establishment's difficulty in determining the overall cause because most doctors are focusing on the pain and are blind to the underlying source of the problem.* However, being unable to accurately diagnose the cause of low back pain eliminates any chance of correcting the underlying problem.

---

* We will spend ample time describing the process of Neuromechanical Imbalance later.

COMMON PAIN GENERATORS IN THE LOW BACK

Without going into detail, we just want you to be aware that there are really only a handful of things that can cause low back pain. You can get low back pain from the disc, the nerve roots surrounding the disc, the spinal cord, the facet (a spinal joint), the ligaments, muscles, fascia, sacroiliac joint, organ referred pain, abdominal aortic aneurysm, cancer, infection, and skin disorders. Now, this isn't the end-all-be-all list, but this list constitutes 99.9 percent of all the possible causes. The list sounds intimidating to the uninitiated, but don't let it bother you. We're about to boil it down even further.

Some of the things on that list are scary but are easy to rule out. And if you have been diagnosed with idiopathic low back pain, then all the scary things should already be eliminated. We're going to assume skin disorders, cancers, infections, abdominal aortic aneurysm, organ referred pain, and, usually, severe spinal cord stenosis have already been ruled out.*

That leaves us with a much more manageable list of possible causes of the pain, which we see every day in our office. They are: the disc, nerve roots, facets, soft tissue (ligaments, fascia, and muscle), and the sacroiliac joint.

If this list still intimidates you, ignore it. The bottom line is that it should be pretty darn simple for a doctor to run through a series of simple tests to figure out which of these, or combination thereof, is creating your problem.

The biggest reason for a lazy diagnosis of low back pain, in our humble opinion, is that as long as the pain is not from cancer, infection, or something requiring immediate surgical intervention, the medical treatment will be the same—pain killers and muscle relaxers. Oh, and you may also be prescribed an

---

* We're making the assumption that these more acute conditions, that require immediate attention, can be easily ruled out by your doctor.

antidepressant just for good measure, since they don't want you to be depressed that you are stuck with back pain for life.

For most medical doctors, what is the point of getting specific about the cause if the treatment is the same? There really isn't one. So they haven't pursued diagnostic skills in this area.

As chiropractors we don't use drugs or surgery, so we are much more motivated to determine what is causing the pain. Also, the source of the pain matters to us because our treatment strategy totally depends on what is causing the pain. For example, if the sacroiliac joint is the primary pain generator and we treat the facet joints, then we won't be successful. So specificity is critical in our approach.

CHAPTER 4

WHAT YOU DON'T KNOW CAN HURT YOU

KEY POINTS

- Muscles and ligaments are rarely the primary source of back pain.
- Facets are only responsible for part of the pain.
- The primary problem behind the majority of low back pain conditions is Neuromechanical Imbalance.

We are going to go ahead and spill the beans here about something else. This is something that even most chiropractors are oblivious to. But it's out there in the research literature, and it has given us incredible results. So we thought we'd share.

The source of pain is even easier to determine than what we let on earlier. *The muscles and ligaments are rarely the primary pain generators.* Do they hurt and ache? Absolutely! But they aren't what triggered the pain. They become aggravated in response to the primary problem.

Again, muscles are not the primary generators of pain. This explains why massage initially feels so great to those with low back pain, but it never gets rid of the pain for more than a few hours or maybe, if you are lucky, a few days. The pain just keeps coming back.

So this little secret means that your low back pain is coming from an even smaller list of possible pain generators. Are you ready to see the list?

1. Discs
2. Facets
3. Nerve roots
4. Scar-tissue adhesions (in the fascia)
5. Sacroiliac joints

Five possible causes are pretty manageable. Do you think it's fair that your doctor should be able to figure out what the problem is from here? We think so.

But we can boil it down even more.

Whenever a disc decays, you can take it to the bank that the facet joints are already negatively affected. This is because the facet joint is dependent on the disc height to keep the appropriate space between its two surfaces. In fact, *studies show that problems in the facet joint always precede disc degeneration (Binder and Nampiaparampil 2009, 15–24).* If the disc degenerates at all, then you can be sure that the facets have already begun to undergo excess friction. Excess friction will lead to inflammation and callouses on the bone (called facet arthrosis). This may or may not cause pain.

The facets are not supposed to carry much weight; they weren't designed for that. Remember, they act as tracks of a drawer that guide motion; they were not designed for weight bearing. When Neuromechanical Imbalance leads to disc decay, weight is shifted off the disc and loaded onto the facet joints. Now they are holding up weight that they weren't designed to handle. It's no wonder why the body creates bone callouses. All that extra friction tells the body that it needs to beef up the facets and make the bone thicker. These bone callouses are referred to as *bone spurs* or *osteophytes*, and they are a normal response to excess stress on the bone. Just as it's normal to develop callouses on your hands from working with tools or weight lifting, bones develop callouses in response to increased friction or load.

Facets only develop these callouses and cause pain if there is something *abnormal* going on. It is estimated that up to 52 percent of idiopathic low back pain is *partly* coming from facets. What is interesting is that only about 4 percent of idiopathic low back pain comes from a single facet *(Binder and Nampiaparampil 2009, 15–24)*.

That means that about half of the low back pain is due, in part, to multiple facet joints. There are two big concepts here. The first is that the *facets are only responsible for part of the pain*. The other is that there is almost always *more than one facet joint involved*.

The explanation is simple, and it's the same for both concepts. There is a mechanical imbalance in the spine causing the weight of the disc to abnormally shift toward the pain-sensitive facet joints.

In addition to damaging the facets, we also know that the disc will begin to decay, as we explained earlier. If the disc decays enough, it can herniate and put mechanical pressure on the nerve root. At the same time the disc is decaying, inflammation is developing in and around the disc itself. What's more, inflammation can also lead to nerve root irritation, giving you problems like sciatica as we explained earlier.

To take this one step further, the bone callouses (bone thickening) of the facet joints can impinge on the exiting nerve roots, therefore leading to another possible reason for sciatica. This is technically called *lateral recess stenosis*.

Are you starting to see the pattern here? Everything we mentioned here originates from the same source...Neuromechanical Imbalance (hmmm...sounds like a theme).

Let's take this concept a step further by stating another constant. If there is pain, there is going to be inflammation.

We know that if the pain has been around for a while, then the inflammation has almost certainly led to scar tissue (which we will explain later). So wherever the pain is coming from, there will be scar-tissue adhesions in the surrounding tissue (fascia). Because of this, fascial adhesions are guaranteed to always be present in chronic low back pain.

With this in mind, what does our updated list of pain sources look like?

Here's the new one:

1. Neuromechanical Imbalance (which leads to disc decay, facet problems, nerve root pain, and consequently, adhesions in the fascia)

2. Sacroiliac joints

Isn't it pretty amazing that 85 percent of low back pain can boil down to two sources?

No?

Wow, the Internet makes it tough to impress anybody anymore; you've seen a one-fingered push-up and a potato that looks like Mariah Carey. So we will just have to push forward like a cheap street performer and give you the whole enchilada.

Drumroll please...

Sacroiliac joint pain is a result of...Neuromechanical Imbalance!

If you are a bit nerdy like us, then your mind was just blown. If not, well, at least we were able to teach you something. Now let's briefly run through an explanation of the sacroiliac joint.

The function of the sacroiliac joint was a contentious subject in the anatomy world for a long time. Until recently, anatomists were saying that the sacroiliac joint *did not* even move, let alone cause pain. However, chiropractors, osteopaths, and other manual medicine practitioners have been successfully mobilizing this joint to relieve pain for decades.* Fortunately, recent research was able to show that the sacroiliac joints do indeed move, so now everybody is on the same page.

When the sacroiliac joint doesn't move correctly, it can cause pain that can show up in the low back, groin, and buttock. This incorrect movement is due to a Neuromechanical Imbalance causing inappropriate loading of the joints, which, in turn, causes inflammation and pain. Nothing new here, but it's still worth mentioning.

So *we have boiled down our list of possible pain generators of low back pain to just one primary cause—Neuromechanical Imbalance.* Like we said earlier, we are going to spend a lot of time on Neuromechanical Imbalance later, so for now just rest assured that your mysterious back pain does have a cause. Even better, there is a way to repair it.

---

* The funny thing about research and theories is that, these days, everybody is doggedly determined to only follow 100 percent research-based practices. While we agree that you would be foolish to ignore research, we also know that the job of future research is to prove currently unproven theories. Simply following research as opposed to leading research limits progress and innovation. Did gravity exist before Sir Isaac Newton "discovered" it? What about ancient Egyptians who prescribed chewing willow bark to cure pain (the substance from which aspirin is made)? If something exists, then it exists—even if we haven't "discovered" it. Even current "facts" that old research has proven are often disproven by advances in technology and better research methods. That's just some food for thought.

CHAPTER 5

HOW DISCS STAY HEALTHY AND HOW THEY BECOME UNHEALTHY

KEY POINTS

- The inner two-thirds of the disc is composed of a nucleus pulposus that is responsible for holding water in the disc.
- The outer one-third of the disc is called the annulus fibrosis, and it serves as the "corset" for the water-filled nucleus (when not damaged).
- Neuromechanical Balance allows body weight to be evenly distributed across and around the disc.
- The disc normally loses some of its plumpness throughout the day but typically reabsorbs water and nutrients during sleep.
- The disc has no direct blood supply, so it must receive its water and nutrients through diffusion from the spinal bones above and below the disc.

- If there is no movement, or if there is an uneven weight distribution from a Neuromechanical Imbalance, diffusion cannot adequately supply the disc, and it cannot be resupplied with water.
- Disc problems can cause nasty shooting leg, foot, and possibly buttock pain, but these symptoms are secondary to long-standing Neuromechanical Imbalances.
- Looking at the spine to find signs of spinal and disc degeneration, sciatica, herniation, or stenosis tells a story about the stressors that we have placed on our body over the years.
- When the spine is out of balance, we can be certain that the nervous system (brain) is also out of balance.

HOW THE DISC WORKS

Two-thirds of the disc is a big, squishy, jellylike substance called the nucleus pulposus. There are molecules in this jelly that absorb water and swell up. Picture one of those little toys you got as a kid that swelled up to ten times bigger when submerged in water. The disc is made up of a bunch of these sponge-like molecules. (Their technical name is proteoglycans.) Their primary purpose is to hold on to as much water as they can so that the disc can be as big and plump as possible. Think about it; if you were a disc, and you had to hold up the spine all day long, would you want to be all dried up and shrimpy, or would you rather be plump and strong like a well-hydrated and well-fed sumo wrestler.

Normal Vertebral Segment
(Front View)

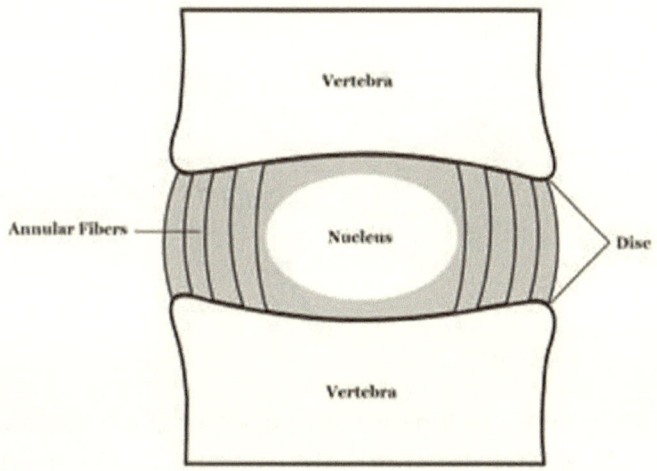

Now that we have an image in our mind of the sponge-like nucleus pulposus, we can talk about the other one-third of the disc—the outer ring, called the annulus fibrosis. This strong fibrous outer ring surrounds the squishy sponge to keep it from escaping. It's a similar concept to a jelly-filled stress ball. Without some sort of strong, yet pliable, wrapper, a jelly squeeze toy would just be a bunch of goop.

The strong, pliable wrapper of the disc is the annulus, and it makes sure that the jelly stays where it belongs—between the vertebral bodies. This wrapper is highly durable, and it has about a dozen layers. Brilliantly, when the body packaged up the disc, it decided to reinforce it with the fibers of each layer lying at a different angle than the next. This pattern provides strength in all different directions, which works well—assuming the body is Neuromechanically Balanced.

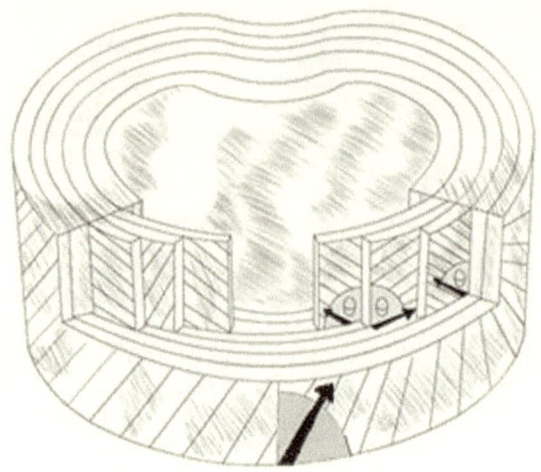

In other words as long as the weight of the body is distributed equally across the entire disc throughout the majority of the day, everything goes well, and the disc is happy. The disc can withstand sporadic bending, twisting, leaning, and stooping because the layered fibers of the outer annulus are highly durable.

However, this supposed strength and resilience of the disc begs the question,

"Why does this tough, shock absorber break down if it's so strong?"

To answer this question, we must first understand a little more about how the disc works and how it gets fed.

HOW THE DISCS STAY HEALTHY

Discs need steady, even pressure applied to them the majority of the time. We must remember that the discs are constantly under a lot of pressure from the weight of the spine and torso when we are standing or sitting, and all of this weight slowly squeezes some of the water out of the spongy nucleus pulposus. This is a normal daily process. To make up for this loss, you lie down at nighttime and unload all of that pressure off the disc. Now the discs can rest, and they can suck some water that was lost back into their sponge. This is why you are tallest in the morning and shorter in the evening.

Normal Balanced Discs

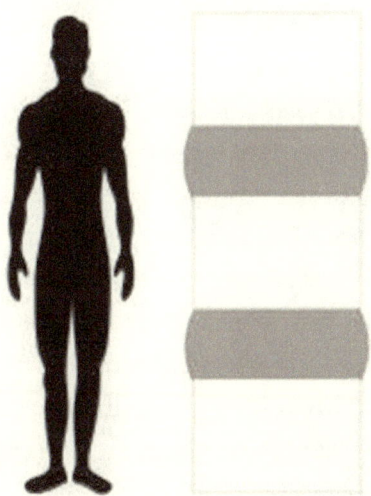

In order to keep the discs their healthy, proper height—full of waterlogged, spongy molecules—the discs must be supplied with water.

Here's the problem.

In the rest of the body, cells and tissues that need nutrients and water get those things from the blood. The blood vessels are the freeways of the body. They deliver all the nutrients we need, including water, to target destinations. Unfortunately for the discs, they are in the backcountry, and the blood-vessel highway system doesn't have a direct route to deliver nutrients or water. But just like all good country folk, they figure out their own way to get what they need. In the case of the discs, they rely on sharing with their neighbors to get nutrients.

GETTING FED

While the discs don't get a direct blood supply, they have a unique system to keep them well hydrated and full of fresh, new spongy molecules (proteoglycans) that hold in this water.

This unique system works through diffusion.

Diffusion is a process where nutrients move from an area of high concentration to an area of low concentration. It's like being on a crowded subway car. Everyone initially starts out jammed together, but as soon as some room opens up, everyone moves to a spot that is more comfortable with more breathing room. To add some numbers to this concept, if twenty people are in one train car, and the next car over is empty, within a minute or two, roughly ten people will leave the overpacked car to go to the empty car. Now there are ten people in each car, nice and comfortable.

This process is exactly how the disc receives its nutrients. The vertebrae above and below the disc get a good supply of blood, and they are willing to share it with the disc.* So if they see that the disc is an empty train car, water and nutrients will make their way in, feeding the nutrient-starved disc.

THE PROBLEM WITH DIFFUSION

To briefly recap, we know that water needs to get into the disc to make it plump and healthy. We also know that the water in

---

* Yes, bones have blood in them; in fact they make blood.

the disc is held in the proteoglycan molecules within the jelly-like nucleus pulposus. So as the weight of the body during daily sitting and standing squeezes some of the water out, causing the disc to shrink, it needs to refuel its nutrients. To make matters worse, some of the proteoglycans get pushed out as well. This is where diffusion comes in.

The surrounding bones and vessels outside of the disc have a lot of water and nutrients that the inner nucleus pulposus of the disc needs. With that in mind, the nutrients should just walk right into the less-crowded train car; but they can't. Of course life couldn't be so simple.

So what's the problem?

The pressure of body weight and gravity is squeezing the spongy disc and not allowing water or nutrients in. Imagine squeezing a sponge in your hand, submerging it in a bucket of water while maintaining a clenched fist, then bringing it back out dry. The sponge will not fill up until you first open your fist and allow the sponge to suck the water in. So diffusion, as it turns out, is only part of the story.

THE KEYS TO FEEDING THE DISC

Movement and sleep are the real keys to getting water and nutrients into the disc. Since the disc is sandwiched and glued to the vertebral bodies above and below, the movement we are talking about is movement of the bones of the spine.

We visualize this as a Chinese finger trap, where you snugly fit one finger from each hand into either side of the papery tube. As you try to pull your fingers out, the middle of the trap sucks in tightly creating a vacuum-like effect. The discs work in a similar fashion.

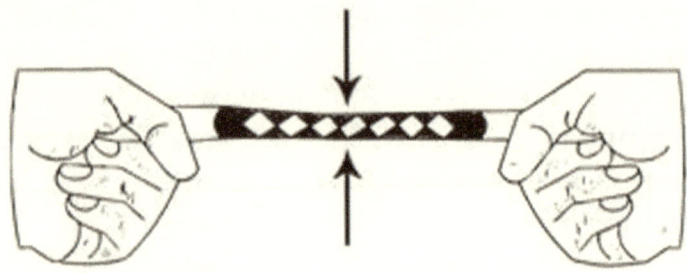

As you bend in different directions, one side of the disc compresses and the other side stretches like the Chinese finger trap, sucking in water and nutrients.

Discs During Movement

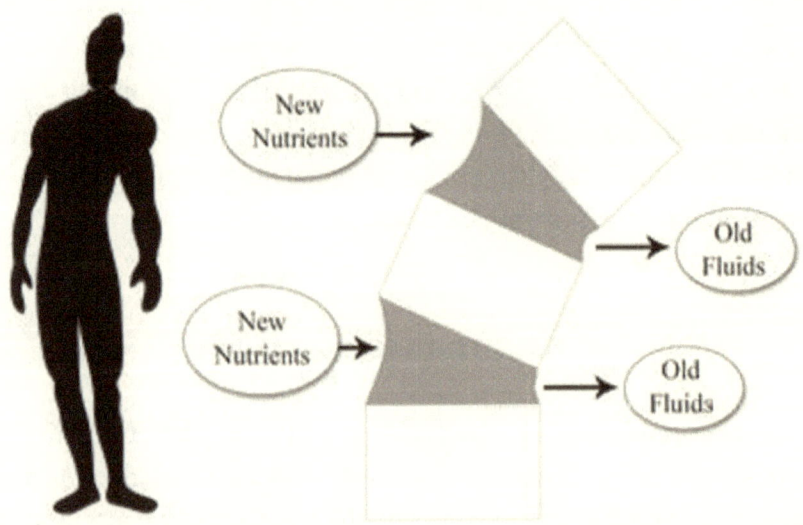

Also, as you sleep, the entire spine is no longer holding up your torso against gravity, which allows the discs to relax and decompress evenly. Lying down creates a substantial drop in intradiscal pressure allowing the spongy discs to stretch and suck in nutrients

Discs When Lying Down

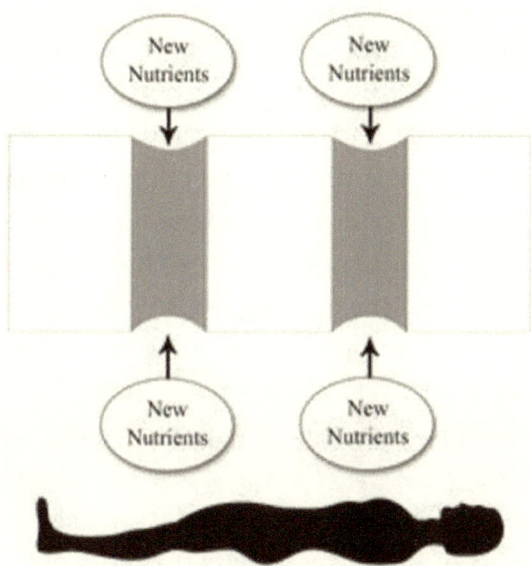

As we can see, it is a combination of spinal movement throughout the day, lying down at night, and diffusion that allows the water and nutrients in the blood-supplied surrounding tissues to make it into the bloodless backcountry of the disc.

Now we can get back to answering the original question.

"Why does this tough, shock-absorbing disc break down?"

LOOKING AT THE BIG PICTURE

We spent a lot of time talking about the disc, and we want to make sure that the big picture is still in focus. *Disc problems (and low back pain) are simply a symptom of a larger Neuromechanical Imbalance in the body.* We thoroughly discussed the steps in which the disc breaks down and the different conditions associated with it (sciatica, stenosis, degenerative disc disease, facet arthrosis, idiopathic low back pain, etc.). This information was necessary to understand why people have back pain.

The information also served a higher purpose. To understand how disc problems cause pain, we were forced to discuss the process behind it. As you discovered, the dysfunction and breakdown of the disc is the way the body is forced to respond when there are long-term *Neuromechanical Imbalances*. The pressures are not equally distributed across the surface of the disc over the long run, and the disc responds by decaying (degenerating and possibly herniating) causing some type of low back pain or shooting leg pain.

All of these problems lead to an even more dysfunctional spine, and *it's easy to see how 71 percent of people with first-time back pain will wind up with a long-term problem*. Unfortunately, it will plague them for the rest of their lives, unless they seek out proper treatment *(Itz et al. 2013. 5–15)*.

What is the *big picture* here? It's not the disc, sciatica, herniation, stenosis, or even low back pain at all. These are all just history lessons; they tell us about our lives and the consequences of the stressors we have placed on our bodies over the years.

We look at the disc like an arborist (tree specialist) studies the trunk of a tree. An arborist studies the rings of a tree and can tell not only how old it is but also the story of the tree's life.

Each tree ring represents a different year and shows evidence of different stressors such as floods, droughts, fires, and infection. The rings also show the good years as well, when there weren't any major stressors. An old tree has been through many experiences, and its story is written beneath its bark.

Our own spines tell a similar story. Looking at the spine allows us to see problems in the bones or discs. It tells the story of how we have handled and accommodated life's stressors. A person who has lived life without polluted air and without any infection, who has never sat, has laughed hundreds of times per day, has slept from sundown to sun up, has eaten a perfect diet with complete nutrition, has exercised, and has drunk lots of fresh water daily, would have a beautifully intact spine. However, as this is almost never the case, our spine shows wear and tear due to the *Neuromechanical Imbalances* caused by chronic stressors. Disc degeneration, spinal arthritis, stenosis, sciatica, disc herniations, low back pain, and so on are all just "rings on our tree" showing how we have been dealing with the stressors in our environment.

These symptoms did not happen by accident; they happened for a reason.

Our low back pain, and the various conditions that can arise related to it, all stem from *Neuromechanical Imbalance*. Neuromechanical Imbalance is a term that encompasses many reasons for the pain you're experiencing. The spine is intimately tied to the brain and nervous system. Therefore, whenever the spine is out of balance, the nervous system is out of balance; and whenever the nervous system is out of balance, it means the spine is out of balance. The spine and nervous system are so interconnected that a problem with one will always cause a problem in the other.

Whenever you have low back pain, or any condition associated with it, you have an imbalance in the nervous system as well.

CHAPTER 6

NEUROMECHANICAL BALANCE

KEY POINTS

- Neuromechanical balance is the state in which the spine and brain are communicating appropriately to one another.
- The brain's desire to be efficient allows us to adapt to our environment, learn new movement patterns, and erase the old, whether they are good or bad.
- The brain requires constant, immediate, and specific signals from the receptors of the spine and muscles.
- The brain uses signals from the spine to not only gather information but to maintain its charge and to remain healthy.
- The brain integrates all of the information it receives and relays signals that include specific locations, commands, and coordination to the muscles of the spine.
- The spine and brain rely on one another for balanced signals in order to carry out appropriate movement.

NEUROMECHANICAL BALANCE

Neuromechanical Balance is a state in which the brain and spine are communicating appropriately with one another.

Just like in any good relationship, communication is a two-way street. Proper communication occurs when the spine sends balanced signals to the brain, and the brain sends balanced signals to the spine. Both the brain and spine rely on one another to function appropriately. The importance of this connection is blatantly apparent in people who have suffered severe strokes.

In these cases the brain is damaged and sends inappropriate, unbalanced signals to the body (and spine) resulting in loss of function. These unbalanced brain signals oftentimes result in a loss of the stroke victim's ability to walk or move (among other things). In these cases the muscles are intact, but the brain that controls them is damaged and cannot send balanced signals. While strokes don't always affect the muscles of the spine directly, this example illustrates how unbalanced or absent brain signals will cause problems with the control of muscles anywhere in the body.

On the other hand, the signals that the spine sends to the brain are equally important. An extreme example of this can be found in people who have broken their spine and have become paralyzed. All of the muscles below the injury are no longer able to communicate and send signals to the brain. This results in a loss muscle function, but more importantly it begins a process of "reorganizing" the brain.

How the brain is organized is dependent on signals it receives from the body. If the brain stops receiving signals from a particular area, then it acts as if that area no longer exists. So, in the case of paralysis, if the brain stops receiving signals from the legs, then not only will the legs not work, the brain will literally erase them from its consciousness.

The brain is extremely efficient, and it doesn't allow wasted space, so anything that isn't used is erased to make room for something else. This is the premise behind the age-old adage, "If you don't use it, you lose it."

This ever-evolving brain-spine (and really, brain-body) connection is what allows us to adapt to our environment on a day-to-day basis. This allows us to learn new movement patterns and erase old ones. This ability can be good or bad.

If we learn something new that is a proper movement pattern, then the spine will send balanced signals to the brain, and the brain will return balanced signals to the spine. In contrast if we learn something new that is an improper movement pattern, then the spine will send unbalanced signals to the brain, consequently leading the brain to send unbalanced signals to the spine. You can see how this is a feedback loop, where the brain depends on the spine and the spine depends on the brain.

What Makes up Balanced Signals?

Balanced signals from the spine must be constant, immediate, and specific to allow the brain to appropriately integrate all the information from the outside world. In other words these signals (which are electrical) are always sending feedback, without delay, about what a specific area of the body is doing. All of this information is required for the brain to appropriately manage movement and spinal stabilization.

In return, the brain is required to send signals with the appropriate location, command, and coordination to the spine and muscles. This will determine which muscles will be performing a task, whether they will contract or relax, and when they will perform their action.

We refer to the signals from the brain to the spine as *neurologically balanced signals*, because they are coming from the brain. Those going from the spine to the brain are called *mechanically balanced signals*.

Together, when these are in harmony, they create Neuromechanical Balance.

Neuromechanical Balance

Brain: The Master Control Center

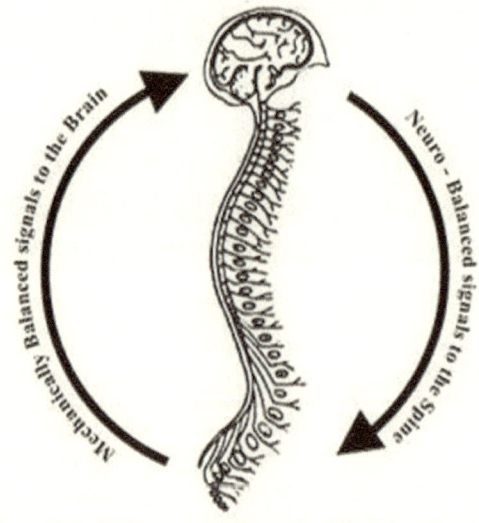

Spine: The Relay and Charging Station for the Brain

STABILITY AND NEUROMECHANICAL BALANCE

We must emphasize the important role that the small muscles of the spine (multifidi) play in stabilizing the spine. If you can recall from the first section, the muscles surrounding the spine are like a stack of pancakes. The deeper ones are intended for stability and maintaining our upright posture, while the ones closer to the top are used for large movements (like bending, leaning, and lifting).

The muscles at the bottom of the stack are called multifidi, and there are hundreds of them. They run down your spine, starting from the second vertebra in the neck, and continue all the way down to your tailbone.* It is the responsibility of these muscles (in addition to others) to stabilize your spine, and they are required to be active at *all* times.

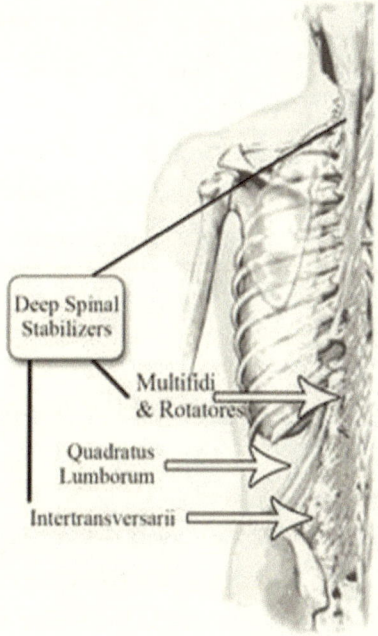

Now that you know what helps to stabilize the spine, we must focus on how these multifidi know how and when to provide stability.

---

* The multifidi are the only muscles that are located atop and across the sacrum.

If you haven't guessed it already, it's the brain's job.

The brain uses special sensors to integrate all of the information from the outside world and tells the muscles where, how, and when their jobs should be performed. To be more specific, the brain will decide which muscle should be doing the job, what it should be doing, and when it should perform a movement.

Together, the brain, spine, and muscles are referred to as the neuromusculoskeletal system.* It's quite a mouthful, but it's just a fancy way of saying the same thing.

Before you get caught up in the word, we simply want you to understand that the brain controls the muscles, which control the movement of the spine and limbs. When these are all working properly, then you have what we call *neuromechanical balance*. However, this is only half of the story.

The brain, although amazing at what it does, must receive constant, immediate, and specific feedback from the thousands of little sensors located throughout the body. These are called the receptors.

These receptors provide a "charge" for the brain. Just as your cell phone must be charged before it can work, your brain must receive a constant charge from the receptors in your body to function properly.

Receptors come in varying types to detect different changes that occur throughout the body; however, they all share the similar function of providing a healthy charge (in the form of electrical messages) to the brain. The main receptors that we are concerned with are the ones that sense mechanical pressure. This is because these receptors are the ones most plentiful in the body, and 60 percent of them just happen to be located within

---

* *Neuro* refers to the brain, spinal cord, and nerves. *Musculo* refers to the muscles, and *skeletal* refers to the bones—hence, neuro-musculo-skeletal system.

the spine. More specifically, they are located within the disc, facet joints, and multifidi. These pressure receptors—mechanoreceptors—are the ones that sense mechanical pressure from movement.

The mechanoreceptors must report their current status, *at all times*, in order to act as a steady charge for the brain. In addition any movement or lack thereof must be immediately reported to the brain *without delay*, to allow the brain to make an immediate decision on how to respond to that information. Furthermore, the brain needs to know exactly *which muscle or joint* the signal is coming from. Simply put, if you're sending signals from your finger, your brain needs to know that it is coming from your finger and not your wrist.

Take a look at the diagram we have provided below.

Neuromechanical Balance

Brain: The Master Control Center

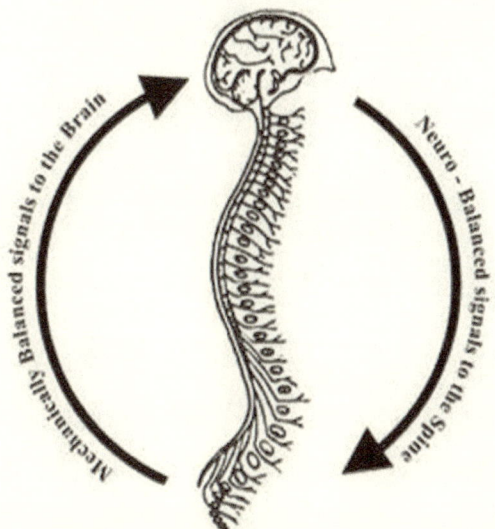

Spine: The Relay and Charging Station for the Brain

The brain receives mechanically balanced signals from the spine. The spine, in turn, receives neurologically balanced signals from the brain about how to move a joint. Said another way, the spine is the relay-and-charging station for the brain, while the brain is the master control center for all functions throughout the body.

That's pretty easy.

Now back to the Neuromechanical Imbalance.

There are a number of reasons why signals going to and from the brain become imbalanced, but we have simplified it for the sake of clarity.

CHAPTER 7

NEUROMECHANICAL IMBALANCE

KEY POINTS

- Neuromechanical Imbalance is the state in which the signals from the brain to the spine, and the spine to the brain, are inappropriate.
- Mechanoreceptors are sensors responsible for sending balanced signals to the brain about joint and muscle position. They are located in your muscles, joints, and fascia.
- The brain relies on constant feedback from the mechanoreceptors to determine the best way to move and to provide a "charge" for the brain.
- Neuromechanical Imbalances are often initially silent.
- The brain creates work-arounds (whether good or bad) in response to inappropriate feedback it receives from the mechanoreceptors.
- When work-arounds are left unattended for too long, there will be a breakdown in the brain-spine connection, and the potential for injury will dramatically increase.

- Multifidi are the deep spinal stabilizers of the spine that are never supposed to "shut off" and are densely packed with mechanoreceptors.
- Inappropriate signals to the brain are called dysafferentation, while inappropriate signals sent to the muscles and joints result in dyskinematics.

Now that you know what constitutes neuromechanical balance, we're going to describe how a Neuromechanical Imbalance occurs. Neuromechanical Imbalance is the state in which the signals from the brain to the spine, and the spine to the brain, are inappropriate. But how do these signals become inappropriate?

To answer this question, we must first take a look at the signals that are being sent from the spine to the brain. As we mentioned earlier, there are mechanoreceptors located all throughout your body that give your brain information about the exact position of all your body parts. It just so happens that the majority of these special sensors are located within the spine.

All of these receptors work together to send signals to specific areas within the brain that provide constant updates about your body's position at any given millisecond. The brain relies on these updates to determine the best way to move. Therefore, the quality of the information that the mechanoreceptors provide will determine the accuracy and appropriateness of the movement.

It's like driving to a new place using GPS. Ideally the GPS will tell you when and where you need to turn with plenty of advance warning. The car's GPS unit sends constant signals to a satellite about where you are in space. The satellite then returns the signal with your location displayed on a map. As long as there is no interruption in the signals, you will know exactly where you are and make it to your destination.

However, if there is any disruption of the GPS signals, then the accuracy of your location will be compromised. At this point you are making decisions based off faulty information, and you are probably going to get lost.

The brain is no different. It relies heavily on the information it receives from the mechanoreceptors to coordinate accurate, balanced movements.

For example, when you bend over to pick up a box, your brain, within nanoseconds, must determine and coordinate a massive amount of information. It calculates how far you need to bend to reach the box, which muscles to activate to grab the box, how much force to generate to pick it up, and which additional muscles need to be activated in order for you to stay balanced. Your brain depends on the mechanoreceptors to give continuous, accurate signals about the location of each body part, so it can safely and efficiently perform the task. Otherwise, you will make a mistake.

MECHANORECEPTORS—THE BRAIN'S CHARGING STATION

As if providing the brain with a constant status update isn't enough, the mechanoreceptors play an even more significant role. They help to keep the brain alive.

Brain cells are unique in that they need continuous activation (charging) to stay alive. Without any stimulation from the various receptors in your body, brain cells will die. While stimulation comes from all of the different receptors throughout the body, the majority of activation comes from the mechanoreceptors. Furthermore, since the majority of the mechanoreceptors are within the spine, the spine plays an immense role in keeping the brain alive.

This is why we like to refer to the mechanoreceptors as the "charge" for the brain. Without them the brain wouldn't receive enough activation to fully "recharge." Although the brain can function without a full battery, it doesn't work as well. It's similar to going weeks without food. Your body can survive, but it is certainly not going to function optimally.

Using the mechanoreceptors as a dual-purpose tool is a brilliantly efficient use of real estate. Since they have to be activated at all times to provide constant feedback about each tiny part of the body, they might as well be used to keep the brain fully charged as well.

Unfortunately, if the mechanoreceptor signals to the brain become disrupted, then you begin to not only lose the ability to make accurate decisions about movement, but you also lose the capacity to fully recharge the brain. This scenario sets the stage for Neuromechanical Imbalance.

NEUROMECHANICAL IMBALANCE– A SILENT BEGINNING

Neuromechanical Imbalances are often initially silent. They slowly and quietly cause the body to become more and more dysfunctional. This is because the brain provides backup plans to compensate for any imbalances that arise. For example, how would your body respond to the challenge of walking with a broken leg?

You would walk around awkwardly swinging your leg in a way that allows you to move with minimal discomfort. Is it the ideal way to walk? Of course not, but your leg is broken and in a cast, so your brain would compensate by creating a work-around.

As the compensation continues over time, the brain begins to memorize your new walking pattern and programs it into the brain. You have effectively taught your brain a new way to walk. The process of reprogramming or rewiring your brain is called neuroplasticity or muscle memory. This new work-around becomes permanent.

Unfortunately, this new walking pattern takes the place of your pre-injury pattern, and you continue to walk a bit awkwardly even after the cast is removed. Unless there was major structural damage, you won't even know that you are walking differently after the cast is off. Your walking pattern will feel normal, yet the pattern is inefficient and won't stimulate the appropriate mechanoreceptors.

This leads to Neuromechanical Imbalance.

Neuromechanical Imbalance

Brain: The Master Control Center

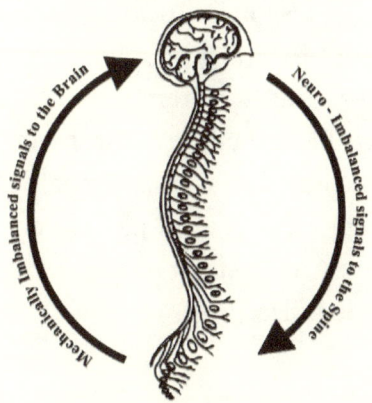

Spine: The Relay and Charging Station for the Brain

The brain becomes efficient at what it does on a regular basis, whether it is Neuromechanically Balanced or not. This means that you can walk, golf, run, bend over, or even comb your hair in a way that is inefficient. One work-around can lead to other work-arounds, and these can accumulate over time. In other words the muscle coordination and feedback from mechanoreceptors can be inaccurate, yet your body will still figure out a way to perform the task.

The only catch is that the compensation will lead to a silent Neuromechanical Imbalance that won't stay silent forever.

When the Neuromechanical Imbalances Make Noise

One of the most common phrases we hear in our office is, "I didn't do anything different; I just bent over to pick up ___, and my back went into a spasm."

This scenario can be quite baffling for not only you but for most doctors. The generic explanation tends to be something to the effect of, "Hey, this is life, and these things tend to happen without any major reason." Oddly enough, this explanation tends to be satisfactory for most people.

Of course you now know better.

It should be pretty clear that the Neuromechanical Imbalance is the culprit. In the previous scenario, the person whose back "went out" for no apparent reason just experienced one of the outcomes that arise when the silent Neuromechanical Imbalance decides to make some noise.

Back Spasms

A great question to explore is why the back goes into a spasm. For that matter why does any muscle go into a spasm? The classic way to explain what is happening is to examine an ankle sprain.

When you roll your ankle, the ligaments and tendons in the ankle joint are damaged. The body needs to heal the damage, so the obvious first step is to prevent further damage from occurring. The body accomplishes this by splinting the area using your muscles like a cast for the ankle, as well as by making the area painful. The body also creates inflammation to speed up the healing process.

So the body uses a muscle spasm like a doctor uses a cast— to protect the damaged areas and allow healing to occur without interruption.

This process makes perfect sense in regard to a traumatic episode like rolling your ankle or a car accident. However, it doesn't quite cut it for the person with back pain that wasn't caused by any apparent injury.

Now, we just explained to you that Neuromechanical Imbalance is the cause of back pain that may have seemed to arise from nowhere. But why then can someone experience such extreme pain or sciatica when there wasn't any problem before? It would seem that there would be a slow ramping up of pain as the Neuromechanical Imbalance increasingly created more damage. Yet this isn't the case...or is it?

OUR AMAZING ABILITY TO ADAPT TO PAIN

Have you ever noticed how quickly you forget what it feels like to sit down? When you first sit down, you feel the hard pressure of the chair on the back of your legs, buttocks, and low back. Yet, shortly thereafter, you tune out the sensations completely. You adapt to it. The same thing happens when you scrape your knee. Initially, you are very aware of the pain and how tight the skin feels, but after a couple hours, you forget about it entirely—until you bump into it, that is.

The brain is incredible at adapting to different types of stimuli. Think about the first few weeks of autumn when the leaves begin to change and the temperature starts to drop to a brisk sixty-two degrees. You now have to grab a coat to go out in the mornings, as well as at night. Fast-forward to the bitter cold of January with temperatures about thirty to forty degrees cooler, where every day is a heavy-jacket day. There may be occasional crazy-warm days when you see everyone outside soaking up the sun in T-shirts and shorts—yet it is only fifty-one degrees! This is a testament to how our bodies can adapt to even extreme temperature changes.

Since our bodies are masters at adaptation, adapting to neurological imbalance is just another day on the job.

The Neuromechanical Imbalance will cause inflammation and damage, but it does so gradually. We know that inflammation will cause some level of pain, but because of the slow change, your body is easily able to cover up the pain so that you can go about your life. Over time there are little hints and signs of problems, but they are so small that you brush them off as insignificant. Waking up a little stiff in the morning is a classic first sign of an imbalance, but it's "normal," so you shake it off. Think about it this way, how often did you wake up stiff or tight as a child? You didn't.

Another early indicator of increasing damage is back soreness. We don't mean the kind you get after a good workout, we are talking about soreness in your low back at the end of a regular workday. Have you ever experienced fatigue between your shoulder blades or around the back of your neck? These aches and pains aren't normal, but they are often blamed on bad pillows, beds, and chairs. The aches and pains are certainly common, but they are not normal for a healthy person. Again, young kids don't complain about these types of things, but adults and teenagers who have been coping with Neuromechanical Imbalance for years do.

Let's explore what's causing the muscle tightness and soreness that we tend to accept as normal or ignore.

THE DEEP SPINAL STABILIZERS

It all comes back to the deep stabilizing muscles of the spine that we introduced earlier—the multifidi. It is their job (along with the rotatores and intertransversarii) to keep the spine in the properly balanced position at all times so the body has a strong foundation. Because there are hundreds of these tiny muscles wrapping the spine, they provide enough strength to hold up the spine against gravity without much extra help from the bigger muscles called the erector spinae.

If you recall, the multifidi are on the bottom of the stack of pancakes, whereas the erector spinae are on the top. In other words, the erector spinae are further from the spine and closer to the skin. The erector spinae are long muscles and span long distances, i.e. from the bottom of the spine to the back of your head. This allows them to act like a crane and tighten up when you bend forward to stop you from toppling over. Basically their job is to allow you to bend really far forward or side to side and then return to an upright position.

Therefore, both the multifidi and the erector spinae have a role to play in keeping you upright against gravity. When you are standing or sitting, the multifidi should be the primary muscles that are firing to keep your spine upright and balanced. But if you bend over, the erector spinae kick in to keep you from falling over, and then they bring you back up.

Back Core Musculature

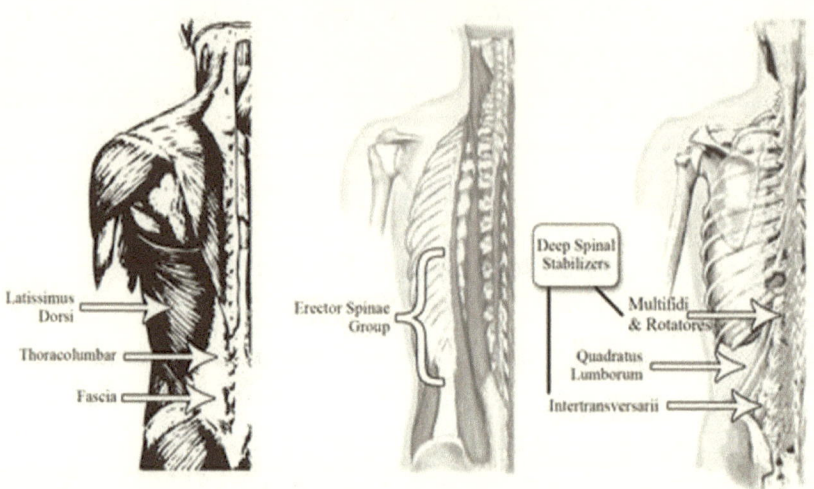

It's important to mention that the multifidi are always working to balance the spine across the discs, even when bending. In other words the multifidi aren't supposed to shut off, even if the erector spinae muscles are firing.

Because these multifidi are always working to balance the spine, they are loaded with mechanoreceptors.

Stability and balance of the spine is so critical that the body wants constant information about the position of each vertebra at all times. As you recall, the body receives this information from the spinal joints (discs and facets) and the deep spinal muscles (multifidi) via mechanoreceptors. As the mechanoreceptors relay information back to the brain, the brain makes decisions about how to move based on that feedback.

Thus, the multifidi play a very important role in maintaining Neuromechanical Balance. They are responsible for maintaining a balanced upright posture, and they send constant signals to the brain about the current status of the spine.

NEUROMECHANICAL IMBALANCE AND THE MULTIFIDI

When the multifidi become compromised, due to inefficient work-arounds, they can no longer send mechanically balanced signals to the brain. Of course if the brain receives imbalanced mechanical signals, then it will respond with imbalanced neurological commands. This imbalance leads to mechanical spinal instability, which is a precursor to spinal injury via disc decay.

As you recall from the *neuromechanical balance* cycle, there must be appropriate signals going into and away from the brain in order for proper movement to occur. When the signals to the brain are inappropriate, the scientific term used is *dysafferentation*. When the brain sends bad signals to the muscles, *dyskinematics* is the result, which is the scientific term for abnormal joint motion.

Since the multifidi are no longer effectively stabilizing the spine, the body is again forced to create another work-around. This time, it recruits the erector spinae to help reinforce the spine and take the place of the multifidi. Now, the erector spinae are firing constantly to stabilize the spine in addition to the multifidi.

Over a long period of time, the multifidi basically shut down because the bigger erector spinae have taken over their job. This is bad news because the erector spinae muscles were never designed to do that job. They don't have the appropriate quantity of mechanoreceptors to give the necessary fine-tuned feedback to the brain, nor do they have the endurance to stay activated at all times. These muscles were only intended to be used occasionally; now they must stay activated indefinitely.

This leads to an even more severe Neuromechanical Imbalance and accelerates the process of disc decay. Furthermore, the erector spinae muscles are reaching the point of exhaustion, which explains why your low back feels tight in the morning and achy at the end of the day.

Ultimately, the disc decay process accelerates and over-whelms your body's ability to adapt to the pain and damage.

This is usually the point when you bend over to put on your shoes and your back suddenly "goes out."

The overworked erector spinae muscles are so exhausted that they can no longer do both jobs anymore. They reach their tipping point and give out—causing an unsustainable stress on the discs, damaging them even more. Many people have been at this point; our bodies are not like the Energizer Bunny that just seems to "keep going and going." Now you suddenly have severe pain caused by a back that is in spasm in an attempt to protect the damaged area.

CORTICAL SMUDGING

You might ask, "What the heck is cortical smudging?"

Cortical describes portions of the brain known as the cortices (plural). The brain has several cortices all serving important functions throughout the body. For the context of this explanation, the area of your brain known as the parietal cortex has a map that is responsible for detecting various sensations that correspond with particular locations within the body.

For example, when someone pokes you in the back, the map in your brain will essentially "light up" in that location to allow you to feel the poke and know its location. The same response would happen if you were poked in your arm, except the brain map would light up in the area corresponding to your arm.

What is amazing about your brain's body map is that it updates and reorganizes, based on new information it is getting from your mechanoreceptors, every couple of weeks. This reorganization can cause changes for good or bad, depending on the feedback it most often receives (or doesn't receive).

How does this relate to cortical smudging?

Each muscle has a distinct corresponding map in the brain that lights up when that muscle's mechanoreceptors are fired. Let's revisit the above scenario when your back "gives out."

Your multifidi are under firing and your erector spinae are over firing. The brain has created a work-around using the erector spinae because the multifidi are sending little, if any, mechanoreceptive charge to the brain. A few weeks have passed, and your Neuromechanical Imbalance persists. You now have established an ineffectively reorganized map.

The map in your brain has combined your multifidi and erector spinae as one. It literally has smudged the two together. This means the brain is no longer able to distinguish a message from the multifidi versus a message from the erector spinae. This malfunction occurred as a result of the erector spinae being fired all the time, allowing those muscles to dominate the smudged map in the brain *(Tsao and Danneels and Hodges 2011, 1–7)*. As a result of the smudging, the messages sent by the multifidi get lost, and the vicious cycle continues.

CHAPTER 8

HOW NEUROMECHANICAL IMBALANCE DAMAGES THE DISC

KEY POINTS

- The disc's health is directly linked to whether or not there are long-standing Neuromechanical Imbalances.
- Neuromechanical Imbalances cannot be reversed unless damage to the disc is also reversed. They work hand-in-hand.
- Uneven squeezing of the disc will create microtears in the annular fibers.
- Lack of movement makes it difficult for the disc to recover its daily water loss.
- Lack of movement can be a result of Neuromechanical Imbalances in and of themselves or a result of trauma.
- Inflammation creates stress in and around the disc and is a normal response to injury that can occur quickly or slowly.
- Scars tell a story of trauma, whether major or minor, and are messy attempts to protect an injury.

- Healthy tissue glides, whereas scar tissue does not.
- The disc can also develop scars.
- Adhesion is another term for scar, and adhesions can be problematic when they are not therapeutically broken up.
- The disc has pain receptors that get "turned on" when decay or degeneration occurs.
- Normal movement that takes water and nutrients to the disc also gets rid of inflammatory molecules.
- An unbalanced disc initiates a downward spiral of microtrauma, inflammation, pain, and scar tissue.

Even though we know that back pain problems stem from Neuromechanical Imbalance, we still need to further explore its effect on the disc. The disc's relationship to the Neuromechanical Imbalance is like the canary in the coal mine.* It is an early indicator that a dangerous problem is present.

As we will discuss later, we cannot reverse the Neuromechanical Imbalance without reversing the damage to the disc. Therefore, understanding how Neuromechanical Imbalance destroys the disc is the first step to restoring balance.

Proper balance of the disc is absolutely critical for its health. Let's get hypothetical for a moment. If you were a disc, and you were given the choice to decide between either not moving all day but having proper balance or moving all day but having

---

* Coal miners would bring caged canaries with them into the mineshafts because the birds were extremely sensitive to toxic, odorless gases. If there was gas, then the birds would die, ultimately warning the miners to evacuate before the gas killed them. The birds were essentially an early warning alarm.

improper balance, you would choose option one without a doubt.

Allow us to explain our rationale. *While movement and balance are absolutely essential for disc happiness and plumpness, an imbalanced load on the disc will destroy it more rapidly than lack of movement alone (Fortuniak et al. 2005, 324–7).*

The tough reality is that you must have appropriate mechanical balance* to have adequate movement. In other words if the vertebrae above and below the shock-absorbing disc are not properly balanced, then there is going to be more stress placed on one side of the disc than the other. Instead of having the weight of the torso balanced nicely and equally across the entire surface of the disc, one side carries more of the weight. It makes sense that loading up the disc unequally is a recipe for disaster, and in fact it is.

The imbalance of weight on the disc pushes the jellylike nucleus pulposus to the opposite side. Let's revisit the earlier balloon example once again. Think of the disc in the following scenario like a water balloon filled with jelly. If you take your two flat hands and evenly squish the balloon between them, the balloon can be pretty strong because it expands outward equally against your hands. However, if you grab the balloon and squeeze it in your fist, it will bulge out wherever it can find some relief, and then it will ultimately pop.

---

* In addition to mechanical balance, adequate movement requires appropriate disc height. A healthy amount of fluid in the disc creates a bigger, plumper disc that maintains proper height. You cannot have proper biomechanics without the disc being both balanced and healthy.

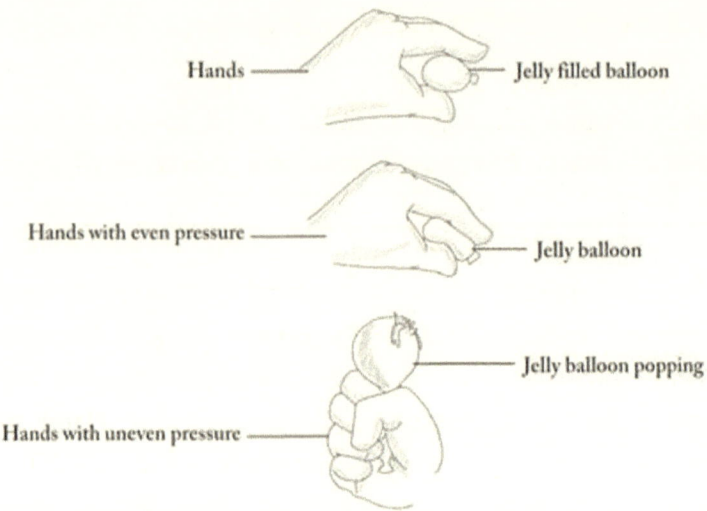

Hands — Jelly filled balloon

Hands with even pressure — Jelly balloon

Jelly balloon popping

Hands with uneven pressure —

The disc likes a nice even distribution of pressure. If the jelly of the nucleus pulposus is squished against one side of the annular fibers unevenly (and too often), then it will start to cause microtears. We will discuss how these microtears lead down a dangerous road later, but first we need to talk about lack of movement.

In a healthy disc, adequate movement of the spine during the day and during sleep at night is barely enough to resupply the nutrients that were squeezed out of the disc the day before. In other words, in terms of resupplying water and nutrients into the disc, there isn't much room for error.

So where does the error come in? One answer is staring us in the face—lack of movement.

LACK OF MOVEMENT

Lack of movement decreases the amount of nutrients that can be sucked into the disc. The disc is a temperamental creature, and if it doesn't move enough each day, the disc will start to lose water and nutrients, even if you lie down and sleep. So, in order to maintain proper disc height, we need the maximum amount of water and spongy molecules in the disc at the start of every day.

Let's say we wake up in the morning, and we have ten drops* of water and nutrients in the disc; it's completely full and happy. Then we go to work or school, doing what we need to do, and at the end of the day, we come home. Even if our spine got lots of good movement, our disc will have undoubtedly lost some fluid (say three drops) but that's OK. We are now left with seven drops in our disc before bed. As we lie down to sleep and decompress our spine, we reabsorb the fluid back into the disc. Then the alarm goes off, and we get up. We should have a full ten drops in our disc again, ready to start the day at optimal disc health.

Unfortunately, for most of you reading this book, this is not how it happens. You wake up with ten drops of water and nutrients in the disc before starting your day. By the time you are home and ready for bed, you have lost a total of four drops (instead of the normal three) because of prolonged sitting, which is detrimental to the disc, and because of imbalanced spinal movement from previous work-arounds. Now you can't wait to lie down when it's time for bed because your back muscles are tired. You currently have six drops of fluid in your disc. Your alarm goes off, and you feel ready to start the day, but now you are starting with only nine drops instead of the full ten, because lying down for sleep only restored three drops. Can you see how this can become a slow downward spiral?

---

* Of course, we have thousands of molecules in the disc, rather than the ten drops of water in the above example. But the process of losing several drops per day gives you an idea of how the slow-and-steady loss of nutrients over a long period of time (months and years) can add up to significant loss of disc fluid and nutrients.

Without balanced, adequate movement of the spine, the discs will not be able to recover all the lost nutrients and fluid each day. Unfortunately, the amount of fluid that can be restored by simply lying down at night is limited. And by the time you notice there is a major problem, lying down all weekend trying to restore lost disc fluid is no longer an option. Now you can see why we say there isn't much room for error.

In addition to lack of movement, the other important stressor on the disc is inflammation.

INFLAMMATION

Inflammation is the body's response to injury, and it is associated with pain, redness, heat, and swelling. Let's start off with an example to illustrate all the components of the inflammatory process.

Everyone is familiar with falling and scratching a knee. The body responds to the injury by calling on its immune system to heal and disinfect the area. The immune system is what keeps you from getting sick and helps heal damaged tissues. The redness and heat around the cuts are there because the immune system requested extra blood to go to the damaged area, making the area warmer and redder in color. The extra blood also transports a larger supply of nutrients that the immune system needs to help heal the cuts faster. The swelling that you see and feel is a byproduct of all the extra nutrients, water, and inflammatory supplies that the blood brought in. In fact any time there is swelling in the body, you can take it to the bank that there is inflammation.

Last, but not least, we have pain. The pain is there to stop you from doing anything stupid, like touching, fiddling with, or hitting your wounded knee again. Your body wants to have the best shot at healing, so it likes to have a protected workspace that will keep the sensitive new tissue and skin protected.

Healing is an amazing thing, and we are fortunate that our bodies orchestrate this impossibly complex task because nobody has been able to fully understand it. What we do know is that, as long as we are alive, we are constantly repairing, replacing, and healing damaged tissues.

What is especially fascinating is that the body even knows when it should do a slow, detailed job versus a deadline-is-due-gotta-get-this-done-today kind of job. Think about all the scratched knees and elbows you got growing up...Now take a look at your knees. There shouldn't be any evidence that you scratched your knee, unless you really gouged it good. You don't have scars because the body realizes that a scratched knee is something minor, and it can take its time repairing it. This extra time will allow the body to do a superb job making your knee look brand new again.

Now think back to a time when things were a little more serious—like the time you decided to catch a wooden boomerang with your forehead, and lo and behold, it split right open. In this circumstance the body doesn't have the luxury of working slowly to repair the damage; it has to stop the leak right now. It does this by bringing in truck-loads of cement and pouring them down heavily as fast as it can. To the body, looking sexy takes a back seat to surviving the trauma, so it does what it needs to get the job done, period. After you are healed, you are left with an ugly scar as a reminder of how much smarter you are after learning one more thing not to do.

SLOW AND UGLY

In addition to healing *slow and pretty* versus *fast and ugly*, there is another way to heal—*slow and ugly*. Let's go back to the example of skinning your knee. So you have skinned your knee, and the inflammatory response has kicked in, beginning the healing process. A nice scab has formed reminding you of what you did, but somehow you manage to trip and fall on the same darn knee, and the scab gets ripped right off. Bummer. It hurts all over again.

This time the swelling and redness are more pronounced, and it's even more painful than the first time you did it. But, just like the first time, a scab forms to stop the bleeding. A couple days go by, and you just can't take how itchy the scab is, so you start scratching around it. The next thing you know, you've picked off the entire scab, and you feel it start to bleed again. Great job, now you get to start the process all over again.

Once your knee finally heals, and your willpower to stop scratching is maxed out, the scab flakes off, and you are left with a bright-pink patch of freshly made skin. The only problem is that the constant interruption of the healing process left you with a scar that you will carry your entire life.

SCARS

Scars all tell a story of trauma. As we saw in the previous examples, the type of trauma that creates a scar can be a major injury or a minor one that isn't allowed to heal properly. When we think of scar tissue, we typically think of a visible mark on the skin left behind after an injury, but it literally goes deeper than that.

Scar tissue is a messy group of specialized tissue that isn't like the original tissue it's replacing. Its purpose is to superglue the injury site back together, and, just like superglue, it sticks to everything around it. So when you have an injury that is really bad, or one that isn't given the chance to heal, the body starts using this superglue instead of slowly rebuilding the normal tissue. The more superglue that is used, the bigger and deeper the scar becomes, and more tissues get stuck together, whether they are supposed to be or not.

Scars are not just on the surface of the skin; they go deep—sometimes all the way from the skin to the bone depending on the injury. Oftentimes scars are underneath the skin, super gluing muscles together. Even fascia, joints, and the protective, lubricating capsule that keeps them healthy, can develop scar tissue. And as you may have suspected, the disc, which is a joint, can also get scarred up.

As we mentioned scar tissue gets sloppily laid down, sticking to everything around it, which in the initial healing phase is great. But, after you heal, having your muscles stuck to your skin, or your skin glued to your joint, poses a problem.

If you have a visible scar, try pinching and rolling it in your fingers while pulling up on the skin. Then do the same thing with the healthy skin on the other side of your body. There will be an obvious difference in how it feels, unless you have had the scar tissue therapeutically broken up.

All the layers of the body are designed to slide smoothly and easily over one another without friction. To be more specific, the skin should slide easily over the underlying fatty layer, and the fatty layer should slide nicely over the muscles. To top it all off, the muscles should slide over one another as well.

All of the tissue layers in the body slide across each other in order to move when they are functioning optimally. If there has been any trauma in the body that led to scarring, you can be certain there are layers stuck together that shouldn't be. The same goes for surgery; you can also guarantee that you will have lots of layers adhered together. In the medical world, we call scars *adhesions*, and they always impair proper function if they haven't been broken up.

Fortunately, scars *can* heal, and the tissues that aren't supposed to be stuck together can be "unstuck" and allowed to slide freely again. We refer to the process of unsticking the layers as *breaking up the adhesions*.

In our office we have found that targeted, high-speed-pressure wave therapy, manual myofascial-release techniques, and tool-assisted soft-tissue mobilization are all great ways to break up the scar tissue. Determining which therapy or combination of therapies we will use to get the best results will depend on how long it's been since the injury, where the adhesions have formed, and the types of tissues involved. But the bottom line is that the scar tissue can be broken up and allowed to move and act like healthy tissue.

It's time to revisit the disc and add in an important concept.

DISC INFLAMMATION

Do you remember how we told you that the disc likes to have even pressure sandwiching it from the vertebrae above and below? Without this balance the disc cannot move properly and, therefore, cannot regain all the water and spongy molecules that it lost during the day. This leads to a loss of disc integrity and to degeneration. By now this concept should be pretty clear.

With that concept fresh in your mind, we can share with you the most cutting-edge research regarding the disc.

Until very recently, scientists believed that discs themselves couldn't cause pain because they didn't have pain sensors. Well, they discovered that they were just plain wrong. Discs do have pain sensors, and they get turned on when the disc decays and degenerates.*

As the disc decays (loss of fluid and water), it gets flooded with inflammatory molecules. Not surprisingly, these inflammatory molecules create inflammation in the jellylike nucleus pulposus. In other types of tissue, like skin and muscle, the highways of blood vessels constantly haul off old inflammatory molecules and bring in new ones (if the body still needs the inflammatory response). But since the disc is in the backcountry without a blood supply, the inside of the disc sits in a toxic bath of inflammatory molecules because it can't easily get rid of them. As you can imagine, the inside of the disc becomes a pretty nasty place. This hot, soupy inside of the disc winds up firing off the pain sensors like crazy *(Krock et al. 2014; Gruber et al. 2012)*.

During the day we lose water, nutrients, and proteoglycans while standing or sitting, and because of mechanical imbalances, we don't reabsorb them all back. The disc decay itself causes inflammation that can't easily escape, causing more and more pain. The poor disc is just sitting there taking one beating after another without relief.

To add insult to injury, the sponge-like proteoglycans are unhappy with all that is going on, and they are dying off in droves *(Zhao et al. 2007)*. They can't survive in the toxic environment that the inflammatory molecules have made in the disc. In response, the body rushes to make more proteoglycans because we need them to hold on to the remaining water in the disc.

---

* Disc decay refers to the process of losing nutrients and fluid from the disc. There is also a build-up of excess inflammation that occurs, and this accelerates the process.

Unfortunately, the new ones that the body spent time and energy creating are too young to function. Even if they were mature enough to function, the inflammation would kill them off too, so it's a losing battle. This process is painful and exhausting, and it becomes a continuous downward spiral.

SCARS AND THE DISC

It is evident that inflammation in the disc is a problem that causes pain, but additionally, it creates scar tissue in and around the disc. As we stated earlier, scar tissue is formed either "fast and ugly" or "slow and ugly." In the case of the disc, scar tissue is usually formed "slow and ugly," due to microtrauma.

Microtrauma simply means that the damage isn't due to a major trauma such as a motor vehicle accident.* It's due to constantly twisting, turning, and bending *with an imbalanced spine*. If the pressure were equal around the disc, then the disc would have no problem with intermittent bending and twisting. But, with an unbalanced disc, the twisting and bending leads to microtrauma, inflammation, pain, and "slow and ugly" scar tissue. These scar-tissue adhesions, in and around the disc, inhibit proper movement from occurring, so the body is forced to compensate with even greater imbalance. You can see how this continues the downward spiral into continuous low back pain.

---

* Many motor vehicle accidents cause significant damage to the body, especially the spine. Even people who don't feel like they are badly hurt often show signs of spinal damage. In fact often people in automobile accidents will lose the normal spinal curvature in their neck, which is a guaranteed imbalance.

CHAPTER 9

DISC DEGENERATION IS NOT A NORMAL AGING PROCESS

KEY POINTS

- Disc degeneration is not normal, nor is it a direct result of old age.
- It is common to see lower lumbar and neck degeneration simultaneously.
- Herniated discs can create shooting leg pain when in the low back, and they can cause numbness, tingling, or shooting pain in the arm or hand when in the neck.
- It is becoming more and more common to find children with disc decay and degeneration.
- Increasing pain from previous injuries in high school sports commonly manifest in the early thirties if not properly cared for.
- When Neuromechanical Imbalances are addressed early in children, they are much easier to restore.

We have previously discussed the process of disc degeneration. Now it's time to call it by its proper name, degenerative disc disease (DDD). Degenerative disc disease is the intense, fear-inducing name for the whole process of how the disc decays and loses its height, in addition to the other destructive processes associated with it.

Most doctors consider DDD to be a normal part of the aging process. However, this process is not normal; there is nothing normal about it.

One of the reasons we know that DDD is not the norm is because of a study done by two Scandinavian researchers. The study was conducted using two hundred random, elderly cadavers (recently deceased bodies). The researchers found that *disc height did not decrease* in the majority of the elderly people examined.

Incredibly, the researchers found that disc height actually increased with old age!

Let that sink in for a moment…The discs, which nearly every medical textbook says will degenerate as we age as part of the normal aging process, are *not* supposed to degenerate. In fact, in the study, the spinal bones actually degenerated before the discs (from osteoporosis), which is why the disc height increased.

Those who suggest that discs are supposed to shrink and degenerate are misinformed and not up to date with current studies. Surprisingly, the Scandinavian orthopedic study we described was published in 1985! More recent studies have since confirmed the original findings *(Twomey and Taylor 1985, 496– 499; Shao and Rompe and Schiltenwolf 2002, 263–8)*.

Think about it this way. If disc degeneration were normal, then we would see fairly equal amounts of degeneration in all healthy discs. Instead, most degeneration is isolated to the low back and lower neck. In fact it's rare to see degeneration in the midback* or upper neck, even in unhealthy aging populations.

In our clinic we often see degeneration and disc decay in both the lower lumbar region *and* the lower neck at the same time. In fact it's not uncommon for patients to have shooting pain in one leg (which comes from the low back) and a strange feeling in an arm or hand (tingling, numbness, or shooting pain), which comes from the neck. These people have herniated discs that are pinching nerves in their low back and neck at the same time.

Researchers have also found these combinations of sensation to be common. They found that 80 percent of people have degeneration in both the low back and neck at the same time *(Matsumoto et al. 2013, 708–13).*

It is our strong belief that it is possible to reach your dying age without any form of spinal degeneration if you have proper Neuromechanical Balance, exercise intelligently, and eat right your entire life. Of course, few people in today's unhealthy world have lived this way their entire life, so it's difficult to demonstrate in research. In other words where are researchers expected to find healthy elderly people for studies?

Perfectly healthy subjects are very hard to find, so they aren't worth hunting for.** Instead researchers typically use the easiest available subjects—the subjects they find in hospitals or colleges who are willing to participate in an experiment.

Think about it: how often are you asked to be in a research study?

---

* The ribs protect the midback, which helps to decrease the occurrence of degeneration.

** For a great book on a researcher who hunted around the world for extremely healthy populations, read *The Blue Zones*, by Dan Buettner. He researched several different areas of the world that had the highest percentage of people over one hundred years of age and came to some fascinating conclusions.

Finding anybody to participate in research studies is extremely difficult, so researchers usually have no other choice than to find young college students (who do not necessarily have a healthy lifestyle) or people in hospitals and other similar institutions. Therefore, it is no wonder why most doctors and health professionals believe degenerative disc disease is part of the normal aging process; they have only studied unhealthy people who have suffered from Neuromechanical Imbalances for years.

We are unfortunately a very unhealthy nation, so we have come to expect these types of problems in our aging populations. It's sad but true. Yet what concerns us most is that people who show signs of disc degeneration and other chronic diseases are getting younger each year. In fact studies are showing that more and more adolescents are showing signs of disc degeneration.

CHILDREN WITH DISC DEGENERATION

This is too big of a deal to skim over, so it deserves its own section. Kids and adolescents with no back pain are showing signs of disc decay, including disc herniations *(Alyas and Turner and Connell 2007, 836–41)*. What is strange is that this doesn't alarm the medical community. Their mentality is, "Well if it's not hurting, then it is nothing to worry about." To them it is just early signs of "normal degenerative disc disease." But now you know better. You know that these youngsters are showing significant signs of Neuromechanical Imbalance.

Because of this attitude from the medical community, there has been very little funding for investigating disc decay in youth. It's aggravating to spend days searching through the medical research only to find so little information about this topic.

Fortunately, we managed to find some very current research from the sports medicine world.

We love sports and sport health research because athletes and coaches care about maximizing human performance, so they fund research that isn't strictly pain based or symptom based. Thanks to these researchers, we have solid research to support what we have been seeing clinically—a rise in disc decay in children. The results were more alarming than we originally anticipated...much more. Here's what we found.

Doctors got together with elite tennis coaches and pulled together ninety-eight elite, junior tennis players who were in top shape, healthy, and had no pain whatsoever *(Rajeswaran et al. 2014, 925–32)*. Half of the athletes were boys, and half were girls all between eleven and twenty-six years old. The doctors took low back MRIs and were stunned by the results. One-third of the kids had one or more disc herniations. Sixty-two percent had disc decay, and 89 percent had facet arthritis...the first sign of disc decay!

They couldn't believe what they found. These were their top athletes, and only 4 percent had no low back abnormality whatsoever. They even found that some of these kids had lumbar fractures. Talk about a lineup for future problems.

In case you forgot, these kids had no pain or problems. Hmmm...do you think we should ignore the fact that 85 percent of our population gets serious low back pain at some point in life? No, it's time to connect the dots.

What these kids are dealing with is not normal aging nor rapid acceleration of normal aging. They have a Neuromechanical Imbalance that is causing rapid, abnormal decay of the disc. Although they are currently pain free, their backs will almost certainly give them problems down the road.

Pain and dysfunction aren't black and white. You don't go to bed perfectly healthy then wake up the next morning in pain and unhealthy. Unfortunately, the majority of the world mistakenly believes this.

Diabetes is a great example of a gradual decline in health. Healthy blood sugar levels should stay between 85–99 mg/dL. Diabetes is only diagnosed if blood sugar rises above 126 mg/dL. Ninety-nine to 126 is a large range, and in order to "get diabetes" you have to be past 126. Once you are beyond that number, you magically have diabetes. Think about this: if your blood sugar level is at 115, are you healthy or diabetic? At 115 you may not have overt symptoms of diabetes, but you are certainly not healthy. You just don't know it yet.

These kids in the study are prime examples of how "healthy" people can have Neuromechanical Imbalance. They are moving toward pain and disease.

How many high-school classmates do you recall that had chronic diseases or bad back pain? Probably few to none. How about after college? Maybe a few. In their thirties? Lots. Do you see the picture we are painting?

You wouldn't believe how many people we see daily who are in their thirties and forties who have back pain, and they tell us that they injured their backs playing high school football or some other high school sport—not collegiate or professional sports, high school sports. For almost all of them, the pain didn't start out as a major problem. In fact, most hardly noticed it while in high school or even when they were in their early twenties. But as they reached their late twenties and turned the corner to thirty and beyond, their previously mild and sporadic pain became more and more frequent and increasingly painful.

The bottom line here is this; kids and adolescents are getting disc decay. This means that they are so neuromechanically imbalanced that they are destroying their discs, regardless of pain. Kids don't stay kids forever, and once their discs decay, it's simply a matter of time before symptoms manifest. And once symptoms show up, they are going to get worse.

Here is one last study we will share before moving on.

This study followed a group of twenty-year-olds *with* low back pain *(Waris et al. 2007, 681–4)*. The researchers wanted to see what the study group's backs looked like on MRI at the beginning of the study and then seventeen years later. They found that, at the beginning of the study, 70 percent of the twenty-year-old participants had decay (without herniation) of one or more discs. This was incredible enough to publish, but the researchers held out and waited for seventeen years and then did a follow-up MRI.

They found that 100 percent of the now-thirty-seven-year-olds had disc degeneration, *and* 76 percent of them had one or more herniations. It is also worthy to note that 10 percent of them had already undergone spinal surgery!

Oh, and all of them still had back pain. Their Neuromechanical Imbalance spiraled downward throughout the years giving them nothing but aggravation and pain.

Hopefully, this gives you the insight you need to have your children checked for imbalance before they wind up suffering the same fate. It's also much easier to restore Neuromechanical Balance in children since there is less local damage to the spine.

CHAPTER 10

COMMON (AND OFTEN INEFFECTIVE) STRATEGIES FOR LOW BACK PAIN

KEY POINTS

- Thirty to 40 percent of spinal surgeries are unnecessary, and 52 percent create even more complications after the surgery.
- Spinal surgery should be the last option of care for back pain.
- If spinal surgery is warranted, do your homework, and look for minimally invasive endoscopic spine surgery options.

Modern medicine offers a wide variety of equally ineffective treatment strategies for low back pain.

As we mentioned before, not many doctors know how to manage your true spinal problems, so they resort to what they know best...drugs or surgeries.

Being a back-pain patient may have led you to become acquainted with several drugs and surgical approaches that, unfortunately, do nothing for your actual problem. However, these drugs do a great job at masking the pain and making you believe that you are better off than you actually are. Here's a running list of drugs that you may be familiar with: nonsteroidal anti-inflammatory drugs (NSAIDs), muscle relaxants, cortisone or lidocaine injections, antidepressants, anticonvulsants. And of course there are different types of back surgeries that are routinely performed.

Let's briefly discuss these latest conventional treatments and therapies, none of which address the true problem.

- Nonsteroidal anti-inflammatory drugs (NSAIDs)— These contain analgesic (pain relieving) and anti-inflammatory properties to treat pain. However, their long-term use is discouraged due to frequent occurrences of adverse kidney and gastrointestinal side effects *(Argoff, Wheeler and Backonja 1998, 833–45; Deyo 1997, 1777–93, Wheeler 2005, 421-52).*

- Muscle relaxants—These are traditionally used to decrease muscle spasms by activating a neurotransmitter (form of messenger) that tells the brain to relax the muscle. However, this class of drugs has demonstrated brain side effects, thus patients must weigh the potential effects against the potential benefits. Needless to say, the muscular pain is secondary to your true problem *(Van Tulder et al. 2003, 1978–92; Malanga and Wolff 2008, 173–84).*

- Spinal injections (such as cortisone or lidocaine injections)—These are local anesthetics, corticosteroids, or other substances that may be directly injected into painful soft tissues, facets joints, nerve roots, or epidural spaces. They, again, do nothing to actually prevent additional damage but provide an artificial Band-Aid on the pain.

- Anticonvulsant drugs—These may be used following failed back surgeries and *may* be appropriate for trial use in specific cases when nervous system structures are symptomatic; however, no studies have addressed whether these drugs will be useful for treating spinal-pain syndromes *(Argoff, Wheeler and Backonja 1998, 833–45; Wheeler 2009, 181–204).*

- Antidepressants—These are commonly used in chronic pain treatment to alleviate insomnia, enhance pain suppression, and reduce painful dysesthesia (unpleasant sensation when being touched). These drugs don't even take away symptoms; they simply make you feel better able to cope with back pain *(Deya 1996, 2840–9, 2849–50; Sindrup and Jensen 1999, 389–400; Watson 2000, S49–S55).*

- *And* back surgeries of various types

As you can see, all of these treatments have dangerous side effects, and most are used for the rest of your life. Most importantly, none of these do anything to address the underlying cause. Many people end up in a perpetual downward spiral of worsening back pain. Drugs and injections offer limited, temporary relief, while allowing the problem to continue to deteriorate. Unfortunately, many people's pain is so severe that they can no longer mask the pain with drugs and become spinal-surgery candidates.

For those who want to get to the source of low back pain and effectively treat the pain for long-term success, you must address the damage to your soft tissues (ligaments, muscles, tendons, disc, and fascia). In addition the imbalances in the brain, spine, and muscles that have created the unsustainable stress must also be corrected. This is accomplished through a two-part approach that first heals the local damage and dysfunction and then corrects the Neuromechanical Imbalances.

SPINAL SURGERY

We have no hidden agenda here. We do not want anyone to have to go through the risks and misery of nonemergency spinal surgery. Our goal is to raise awareness that there are less-dangerous options that are worth considering before having a procedure done that can never be undone.

However, even in our clinic, we occasionally see people whose discs are so severely damaged that they are beyond our capacity to restore. In these instances surgery may be warranted and can be beneficial. To be clear, if you have not done all the researched therapies in this book, or have not been to a health-care professional who employs these therapies, then surgery may not be warranted. *We strongly recommend that you at least try spinal-decompression therapy before considering any type of low back surgery.*

So what is the problem with most nonemergency spinal surgeries (especially spinal fusion) for the treatment of low back pain, stenosis, sciatica, and disc herniation?

Consider this...

In 2012, research was published in *Spine* (a prestigious research journal for spinal surgeons) that reported on the outcomes and dangers of low back surgery *(Lee et al. 2012, 197–206)*. They reported that the complication rate was 52.58 percent within a two-year follow-up. That means that *just over half of all back surgeries had major or minor problems due to the surgery itself.*

What is astonishing is that the researchers who published that study were top-notch orthopedic surgeons sharing their own clinic's personal data. They weren't afraid to share those statistics because they understood that those numbers reflect the current norm, and, more than likely, their clinic has a significantly lower complication rate than most others out there.

It's hard to believe that it has become acceptable to treat low back pain with a surgery that is known to lead to complications more than 50 percent of the time.

While it is admirable that these surgeons shared their personal complication rates with other surgeons, you can rest assured that they neglected to include that information on their practice's website. In fact that particular article was excluded from the list of published research papers that they share with potential patients. Could you guess why? While a 52 percent complication rate may be good for most spinal surgeons, it doesn't instill much confidence in the minds of people considering back surgery—nor should it.

To really understand how dangerous back surgery is, you need to put it into perspective with other types of surgeries. General surgery and trauma have a combined complication rate of 32.3 percent. Cardiothoracic surgery, which is chest and heart surgery, has a 26.9 percent complication rate. And vascular surgery has a 42.4 percent complication rate.

Are you starting to realize why back surgery should be a last resort?

Another alarming statistic comes from the prestigious Dartmouth Institute of Health Policy. They suggest that 30 to 40 percent of back surgeries are completely unnecessary *(Smith 2014).* These facts are disturbing. When other medical doctors and surgeons are saying there is a problem, then there is a problem.

Here are some more disturbing facts.

In October 2013, the *Washington Post* published yet another critical article on spinal surgery titled, "Spinal Fusions Serve as a Case Study for Debate Over When Certain Surgeries Are Necessary."

Here is what they found in Florida alone.

1. Fusions increased sixteen-fold from 969 in 1992 to 15,599 in 2012. (This is an insanely rapid increase in *any* procedure, let alone one as highly invasive as this surgery.)

2. Average case cost nearly tripled from $40,996 to $111,662. (There is no reasonable explanation for this exorbitant rise in costs.)

3. The hardware used in low back surgeries also rose from $12,548 in 1992 to $50,570 per case in 2012—again, an unreasonable rise in costs.

And to top it all off…

4. Half of the 15,599 back surgeries were deemed of questionable necessity. Yes, you read that right…50 percent.

Money is, unfortunately, steering the ship of the American medical spine industry, despite the research and spine surgery guidelines to the contrary.

With all of that said, if you are in the unfortunate circumstance where you do need surgical intervention, we strongly recommend that you do your homework.

At the time of this publication (2014) our local community in California has seen a tremendous rise in spinal fusions (cages) that reflect a similar trend to the Florida numbers shown earlier. Spinal fusion is *not* a new technique, nor is it a good one. Do not get a spinal fusion unless you literally have no other choice (and other nonfusion surgeries failed you). It's highly invasive, meaning they cut you open and screw a huge cage into your spine to completely stop it from moving.

It has been suggested that the reason surgeons are using this older technique is because they have figured out how to make more money doing it instead of developing other, more cost-effective and better, procedures. We suggest that you read the full *Washington Post* article that we cited earlier if you want more information on how some surgeons are abusing the system at the expense of their patients.

PRP Therapy

If other options have failed, and you're on the verge of opting for surgery, PRP therapy should be explored. Platelet Rich Plasma (PRP) therapy is a fairly recent non-surgical treatment for low back pain that is showing a lot of promise. PRP is described as a simple procedure that begins with a small amount of blood drawn from the patient. The patient's blood is then spun until the platelet rich plasma (PRP) separates from the rest of the blood. The doctor then injects the PRP into the injured area of the patient.

Platelets secrete growth factors that stimulate repair of tendons, ligaments, muscle and cartilage. Concentrating the patient's own platelets and then re-introducing the platelet rich plasma into the damaged area can accelerate healing, in theory.

PRP has been used in dental and cosmetic surgery since the mid-1990's. It began gaining traction in the sports medicine field due to its apparent ability to speed up recovery from knee, shoulder and elbow injuries. Recently, physicians are beginning to use PRP therapy for low back injuries with encouraging results.

Dr. Dwight James, a physician in Porterville, California states, "I have been getting good results using PRP for hip and knee pain and have recently started using PRP therapy for low back injuries with very good outcomes." For his contact information, refer to our Patient Resource section in the back of the book.

CHAPTER 11

OUR TWO-PART APPROACH FOR THE TREATMENT OF LOW BACK PAIN

You are now ready to learn about our two-part approach used to heal your low back condition. As mentioned in chapter one, our treatment consists of two parts. Part one will heal the damage in the passive systems of the body, and part two will restore the Neuromechanical Imbalance that caused the damage in the first place. First let's briefly review and expand upon your understanding of the Neuromechanical Imbalance.

Earlier (in chapter one) we told you that the ultimate cause of Neuromechanical Imbalance is chronic stress; now it's time to elaborate. The chronic stress cycle diagram illustrates the following points.

1) Chronic stressors such as inflammatory diets, loss of sleep, poor breathing, bad posture, prolonged sitting, and other environmental and psychological stressors cause a disruption of normal brain function. This disruption is called autonomic imbalance (dysautonomia) and is an imbalance of the brain's autonomic control center. Stress physiologists call this process *allostatic load*. These different terms may seem confusing, so we simply call it *Neuro-Imbalance*.

2) Neuro-Imbalance, in turn, leads to a wide range of conditions and dysfunctions such as systemic inflammation, fatigue, diabetes, cardiovascular disease, autoimmune disease, and neurodegenerative disease, to name a few. In addition neuro-imbalance will always cause mechanical imbalances of the spine. As mentioned earlier 75 to 80 percent of all chronic diseases can be attributed to neuro-imbalance.

3) Mechanical imbalance (dyskinematics) leads to spinal decay—damage to the passive system, which includes disc degeneration, facet arthrosis, fascial scarring, etc. The process of neuro-imbalance leading to mechanical imbalance is, of course, Neuromechanical Imbalance.

4) The consequences of damage to the passive structures from the mechanical imbalance, as well as the chronic conditions caused from the neuro-imbalance, act as internal stressors (stress created inside the body) that feed back into the brain reinforcing and amplifying the neuro-imbalance.

This entire process is a vicious cycle—a feedback loop that will continue even when the original chronic stressors are removed or eliminated. This self-perpetuating feedback loop is called the chronic stress cycle. Once the internal stressors become established (i.e. diabetes, cardiovascular disease, Neuromechanical Imbalance, etc.) they continue to wreak havoc on the brain's autonomic control centers and disrupt autonomic balance. In other words once this process begins, it will continue until interventions are introduced to break the cycle.

You will learn more about the chronic stress cycle in part three. Our patients find that this diagram (located on the next page) is enlightening because it helps them understand the relationship between stress and pain. For example, getting in an argument with your boss (psychological stress) can cause immediate back pain just as eating the wrong foods (increasing systemic inflammation) can also—within hours—increase your back pain.

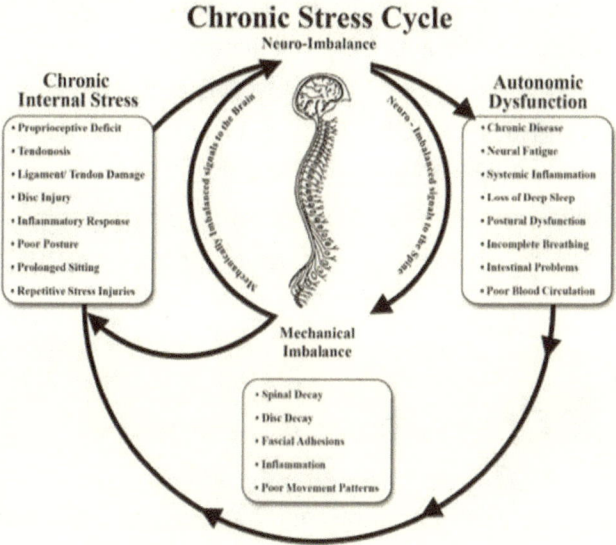

Chronic Stress Cycle
Neuro-Imbalance

Chronic Internal Stress
- Proprioceptive Deficit
- Tendonosis
- Ligament/ Tendon Damage
- Disc Injury
- Inflammatory Response
- Poor Posture
- Prolonged Sitting
- Repetitive Stress Injuries

Autonomic Dysfunction
- Chronic Disease
- Neural Fatigue
- Systemic Inflammation
- Loss of Deep Sleep
- Postural Dysfunction
- Incomplete Breathing
- Intestinal Problems
- Poor Blood Circulation

Mechanical Imbalance
- Spinal Decay
- Disc Decay
- Fascial Adhesions
- Inflammation
- Poor Movement Patterns

As you can see from this diagram, a two-part approach is necessary. The damage to the passive system that is caused by the mechanical imbalance must be directly addressed, and the neuromechanical balance in the active system must be restored.

And here's where things get interesting. By addressing the active system, we are not only restoring balance to the spine, we are also restoring balance to the autonomic system, which affects all systems of the body and will have a major impact on a person's overall health and vitality.

PART ONE—TREATING THE PASSIVE SYSTEM

In order to treat the passive system, we must first be able to measure it. We do this the same way most other doctors do. We begin with a detailed history followed by an observation of gait, posture, range of motion, movement analyses, and specialized orthopedic tests. In addition we use X-ray, CT scans, or MRI when required. The objective is to accurately locate and assess the damage and pain generators. By utilizing the most proven tools and therapies available, our goal is to heal the damaged areas as quickly and efficiently as possible.

The following are the most common structures damaged from mechanical imbalance and the therapies we have found most useful.

Scar-Tissue Adhesions

These are protective barriers that have formed as a result of injury or inflammation. They can spread, entrapping nerves, cause pain or numbness, and limiting normal motion.

Effective therapies we use are…

- Manual and instrument-assisted myofascial-release techniques
- Targeted high-speed-pressure wave therapy

Facet Damage

As you may recall, these facets are the sensitive joints of the spine that guide motion and can become inflamed or thickened with arthritis (called facet arthrosis). Facet damage can generate pain as well as entrap nerves.

Effective therapies we use include…

- Spinal mobilization
- Super-pulsed cold laser

SACROILIAC JOINT DYSFUNCTION

Like facet joints, these are sensitive joints that help guide motion and can become inflamed and arthritic.

Effective therapies we use are...

- Super-pulsed cold laser
- High-frequency percussion

LIGAMENTOUS INJURY

This damage to the leather strappings that hold bones together is a result of acute or repetitive stress or blunt trauma. When they are injured, ligaments can produce pain and cause further instability to the spine.

Effective therapies we use are...

- Targeted high-speed-pressure wave therapy
- Elastic therapeutic tape
- Super-pulsed cold laser

DISC INJURY

As we have discussed in earlier chapters, the disc is always involved with any chronic low back pain condition. Any successful treatment must decrease inflammation and decompress the disc.

Effective therapies we use include...

- Flexion-distraction techniques
- High-frequency-pressure wave therapy
- Super-pulsed cold laser
- Spinal-decompression traction therapy

We have found spinal-decompression traction to be an extremely valuable therapy when working with patients who have severely decayed or damaged discs. In fact this is the most aggressive nonsurgical therapy available. Because of its importance, it deserves its own section and will be covered in the next chapter.

While we are working on healing the damage to structures in the passive system, it is essential to restore Neuromechanical Balance to stop the ongoing damage.

PART TWO—RESTORING THE NEUROMECHANICAL SYSTEM

As you may recall, Neuromechanical Imbalance is a pathological process where neuro-imbalance leads to mechanical imbalance. The same principles that applied to the passive structures apply to neuromechanical balance. We first need to measure and quantify the Neuromechanical Imbalance before we can work to correct it.

As we mentioned in chapter one, measuring the autonomic system and evaluating Neuromechanical Imbalance wasn't previously practical in the clinical setting. Practitioners treating this condition had to rely on vague symptomatic improvements to determine the effectiveness of their treatments. Due to the advances in technology available to the practitioner, we can now accurately measure autonomic imbalance—and thus Neuromechanical Imbalance—with precision. This new availability has allowed us, and other practitioners, to evaluate the effectiveness of treatment interventions and to refine our approach.

Some of the tools we use to measure Neuromechanical Imbalance include heart-rate variability, functional neurological testing, skin conductance, tissue perfusion, neurological stability assessments, and surface EMGs.

Based on testing and patient outcomes, the following therapies have proven to be highly effective in restoring neuromechanical balance in our office.

- Targeted unilateral spinal adjustments
- Dural stretching techniques
- High-frequency percussion therapy
- Active therapeutic movements
- Functional neurological interventions

The therapies we use now are simply snapshots in time that can be used to measure progress. The underlying principle that makes this method so effective is the two-part approach. The ability to accurately measure progress allows us, and other practitioners, to continually evolve and improve our therapies with better clinical outcomes.

ONCE THE PAIN IS GONE

Alleviating pain is not our end goal; it is just the beginning. Don't misunderstand; it is important to remove pain because chronic pain, in and of itself, can create Neuromechanical Imbalance (*Slosberg 2009, 27(2)*).

In an ideal world, in the absence of chronic stress, completely restoring neuromechanical balance is possible. However, as you will learn more fully in part two, completely eliminating chronic stress in this day and age is practically impossible. Once a person's Neuromechanical Balance is optimized, he or she will likely require periodic "tune-ups" to maintain optimal balance.

In other words it will take time to rebalance the body even when the pain is gone. While being pain-free is great, it's only the first step to resolving the bigger issue—the Neuromechanical Imbalance.

CHAPTER 12

SPINAL-DECOMPRESSION TRACTION

Key Points

- Spinal-decompression traction restores the disc with water and nutrients necessary to heal the disc as well as flushes the inflammation out.
- Decompression therapy must be continued beyond the cessation of pain to ensure the disc is completely healed.
- The disc typically takes about ten weeks to adequately heal.

As we promised we will now speak directly to those of you who are experiencing severe low back pain accompanied with sciatica. This type of pain definitely requires a bit more attention, and here's why.

You have had the Neuromechanical Imbalance for so long that it has affected your poor spongy disc, and now it is requiring more direct and immediate attention.

An injured disc looks like a war zone, complete with collapsed buildings, trash-covered streets, massive casualties, and continuous attacks. It's definitely not what you imagine a healing environment to be. So we have to do something to change the environment of the disc and turn it from a war zone into a tropical paradise.

Now to do something this drastic requires an intelligent plan. So what is our plan?

We imagine this process to be like garage cleanup. It all starts with getting rid of the trash and clutter and figuring out what you want to keep. Getting rid of the junk can be an intensive process, and it requires a lot of energy, so we need to bring in some outside help. Fresh, new molecules of oxygen, water, and proteoglycans are a good start. But we know that our disc can't easily bring those in, due to the downward spiral that the Neuromechanical Imbalance created.

It would seem that some sort of intervention is required. Getting rid of the bad and bringing in the good has been a real problem until the invention of several technologies and approaches that works to "pump" the disc, clean up the inflammation, and speed up the healing process. These options are the same as the ones used for low back pain with no shooting pain, but with the addition of one particular therapy—spinal-decompression traction.

How Spinal-Decompression Traction Works

Even though we covered spinal-decompression traction in the passive structure treatment section in the last chapter, we feel it's important to give this incredibly effective therapy its own chapter. In the last few years, spinal-decompression traction has proven, in our clinical experience, to be the most effective nonsurgical therapy for severely damaged discs.

As we know, the disc requires movement to create a vacuum inside of the disc, where it sucks in water and nutrients. But due to Neuromechanical Imbalances, the movement and restoration of disc fluid becomes inadequate. Therefore, we have to do something powerful that can draw nutrients back into the disc and flush out all of the bad, inflammatory molecules that have been trapped inside the disc. This is where spinal-decompression traction comes to the rescue.

Spinal-decompression traction comfortably separates the discs, nonsurgically, using a machine that basically stretches your torso. This stretching draws healthy fluid into the disc by separating the lumbar vertebrae. It sucks in fluid just as pulling your fingers in opposite directions shrinks the center of a Chinese finger trap; a vacuum effect is created. Therefore, by stretching out your torso, you can force fresh fluid and nutrients into the disc. But there is more to decompression traction than just this.

If stretching the spine and separating the vertebrae were all the traction did, it would be only a fairly effective therapy.

Why is this?

Although separating the vertebral bodies and sucking in a bunch of nutrients would feel great while the stretch was applied, after the session was over, there would be too much extra pressure in the disc. Once you stood up and put weight back on the disc, all that fluid would push right into the torn annular fibers and would further exacerbate any herniation (bulge) present. That would be unpleasant, to say the least.

Furthermore, no beneficial healing could occur because you would have aggravated the damaged disc—increasing the inflammation. Plus the same old inflammation would still be present because the trash was never taken out. The type of therapy just described is *ordinary traction*, which is night-and-day different than decompression traction.

Ordinary traction just pulls for an extended period of time and then releases the weight when you are done. This leads to the problem just described above. It is also less effective at separating the vertebrae—which is necessary to create the vacuum effect—because the table creates too much friction and loses the pull. Adequate pull is necessary to create the vacuum effect within the disc. Modern decompression tables are engineered to pull more directly on the spine creating a precise distraction on the intervertebral disc while overcoming the previous problems of friction.

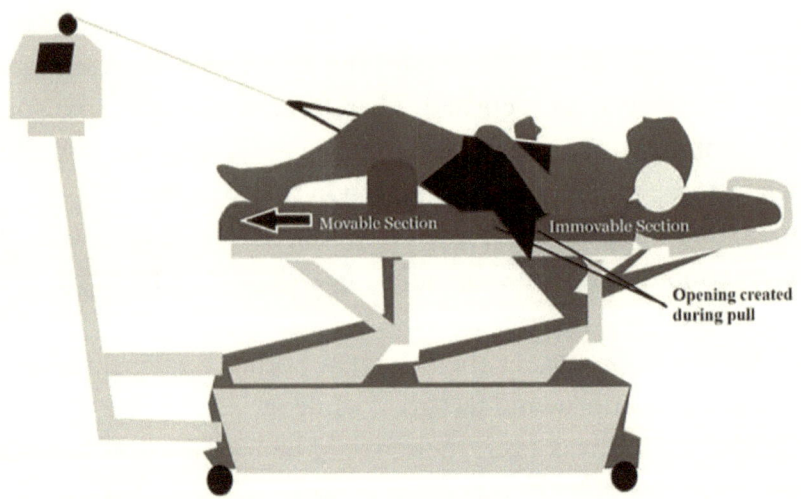

More importantly, the biggest failure of ordinary traction is its inability to remove the inflammatory molecules, and those molecules must be removed for the necessary healing to occur inside the disc. Fortunately, those who developed spinal-decompression traction machines were well aware of this need and created an elegant solution. The solution was to pump the disc.

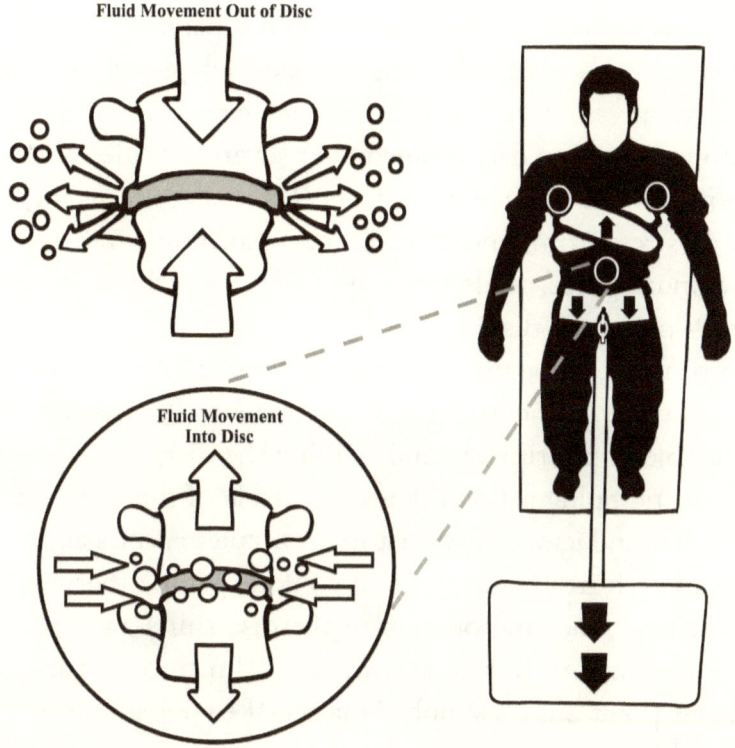

Pumping the disc separates the vertebrae to draw nutrients in and then compresses the vertebrae to expel the water and trapped inflammatory products out. It's like starting with a glass of dirty water and pouring half of it out, then adding clean water until it's full again. What you are left with is a *diluted* glass of dirty water. But if you continue to do this over and over again, you will eventually wind up with a clean glass of water. Pumping the disc achieves this same effect. We are "pouring out" some of the bad disc fluid and then sucking in the good. Over time, the inside of the disc will have very few inflammatory molecules, yet it will have lots of fresh nutrients and water—the ideal healing environment.

Decompression traction has specific computerized algorithms (programs) that alternate between separating and relaxing the lumbar spine, achieving the desired pumping effect. The decompression traction developers have compiled these algorithms from the data gleaned over several decades of treating thousands of disc-injury patients. These algorithms include ratios of stretch time, hold time, and relaxation time, as well as how much force needs to be applied to actually do what is needed—pump the disc.

Fortunately, doing traction this way doesn't leave the disc full of excess water and nutrients that it can't handle. Instead, like the example of pouring out and refilling the dirty cup of water, the gentle pumping action dilutes the inside of the disc removing the pain-inducing inflammatory molecules and washing the disc clean with fresh nutrients that couldn't get in otherwise.

Over time, the environment of the disc shifts away from a nasty inflammatory war zone toward a calm tropical paradise. From this point on, it's simply a matter of time before the disc can fully heal itself, as long as the treatments are continued.*

One of the downsides of decompression traction is that it often works too well. It gets rid of the pain pretty quickly (with significant improvements within several weeks), and because of this people occasionally quit their treatment too soon. They believe that they are healed since the pain is completely gone. Well the problem is that although the pain is gone, it doesn't mean the disc is fully healed.

In fact it takes about ten weeks for the disc to adequately heal. Stopping the treatment after a few weeks because the pain is

---

* Full restoration of the discs is not always possible; it depends on the severity of the damage. But usually enough healing can occur to relieve back pain and shooting leg pain. Research shows that 71 percent of patients get full resolution of pain with decompression traction alone.

gone is not wise because there has not been enough time for the disc to fully heal, and the problem is likely to return. According to the research, it takes about twenty sessions before the disc is adequately healed, and we have found this to be true in our clinic as well *(Gose et al. 1998, 186-190)*. As a general guideline, expect it to take two to three months before decompression is complete and you can get completely back into strenuous physical activity. Think of it this way, it took years for your discs to become this severely damaged, so be patient. It's going to take some time to heal.

WHAT DO STUDIES SAY ABOUT SPINAL-DECOMPRESSION TRACTION?

In an effort to be completely transparent, we want to be careful not to mislead anyone. Spinal-decompression traction is extremely effective, but it does not help 100 percent of patients with severe disc decay or disc herniations. We will share with you the results of a research study done reviewing its effectiveness.

The study examined seven hundred seventy-eight people with damaged discs (degeneration and/or herniations) and constant back pain. The average person in this study had these problems for over three years. These people were obviously desperate for help *(Gose et al. 1998)*. They were treated using spinal-decompression traction for about twenty treatments on average, and the results were impressive.

Seventy-one percent of patients had complete recovery, meaning their back pain and symptoms were completely gone. We repeat: after three years of constant misery, their back pain was gone.

To give perspective concerning clinical research, if a drug is found to be 30 percent effective for a condition, you just struck gold. If you are around the 50 percent range, you now own the market. So 71 percent is an incredible success rate.

However, 71 percent is not 100 percent even though it is an excellent outcome rate.* This option looks especially positive when comparing it to your other options—spinal surgery or drugs.

Now that you have a better understanding of Neuromechanical Imbalance and its relationship with the spine, it is time to expand our focus once again.

Up to this point, we have explained how the brain-spine connection works and how the brain and spine rely on one another to maintain balanced signals. We have also described what happens when there are imbalanced signals and how those signals lead to Neuromechanical Imbalances.

Aside from examples of trauma, we have chosen to keep our explanation of chronic stress brief for the sake of simplicity. Now, however, we are going to dig deeper into the causes of the chronic stress cycle and its affect on your health.

Part two of the book is designed to help you understand what chronic stress is, how it's created, and its implications. After attaining a general understanding of chronic stress, you will easily be able to see how it feeds into brain imbalances leading to chronic diseases and spinal decay. In other words we all

---

* We believe the outcomes in our clinic are better than published research because of our two-part approach that treats not only the damage, but also the cause of the underlying damage (removing the Neuromechanical Imbalance as well as treating the disc directly).

have chronic stress to thank for throwing our bodies off tilt and leading us down the path of disease and pain.

Without further adieu, let's learn about this stress response.

Part II

The Chronic Stress Cycle

CHAPTER 13

THE STRESS RESPONSE

KEY POINTS

- The nervous system is divided into two parts. The *voluntary* nervous system is in charge of things you consciously control like movement. The *involuntary* nervous system is in charge of things you don't consciously control like blood pressure and digestion.
- The involuntary nervous system is split again into two divisions—the *sympathetic* and *parasympathetic* nervous system. The sympathetic nervous system is responsible for *effort and activity,* whereas the parasympathetic nervous system is in charge of *recovery and healing.*
- Our bodies were designed to operate optimally with more parasympathetic (rest and recovery) activity. However, different stressors (physical, mental, chemical, etc.) cause people in today's society to operate predominately in sympathetic mode (effort and activity).
- Fight or flight (extreme activation of sympathetic response) is the body's defense mechanism, designed

to save you from being eaten. It was never designed to be frequently triggered.

- When the sympathetic nervous system is dominant, it becomes a major burden on the body and leads to disease and spinal decay.
- It doesn't matter what the stressor is, the stress response is surprisingly consistent. Your body reacts the same way if you are running from a bear or giving an important public speech (racing heart, sweating, tunnel vision, anxiety, digestion stops resulting in a stomachache, etc.).
- *Neuro-imbalance* (autonomic imbalance) occurs when the stress response is activated too often, and the body stays in a sympathetic state without fully returning to the parasympathetic state.
- Physical stressors can be either acute or silent. The *silent physical stressors* are the ones that are the most dangerous to our health because most people don't know what they are.
- Acute stress is good for the brain and actually improves the brain, which in turn maintains neuro-mechanical balance.
- Frequent stressors can lead to a *low-grade, chronic stress response*. This is when you are exposed to some type of stressor on a continual basis. *This can even be due to something as common as chronic poor sleep.*
- A low-grade chronic stress response is typically due to silent stressors that never allow your body to consistently return to a parasympathetic state. *This is the culprit for almost all chronic diseases.*

THE INVOLUNTARY NERVOUS SYSTEM

The first concept you need to understand is the division of the nervous system. Very simply, the human nervous system is broken down into two parts: the voluntary nervous system and the involuntary nervous system. It works just like it sounds. The voluntary nervous system (aka somatic nervous system) consists of things you can consciously control, like raising your arm, running, smiling, and swallowing food. The involuntary nervous system (aka autonomic nervous system) consists of things your body does on its own—for example digesting food, adjusting heart rate, control of internal organs, etc.

There are a few functions shared by these two systems, namely breathing and blinking. Your body will keep you breathing and blinking without you thinking about it, but you can consciously control these functions at any time as well.

The involuntary (autonomic) nervous system is the part that we are going to focus on. Coincidentally, it is also divided into two parts—the sympathetic nervous system and the parasympathetic nervous system. While these two halves oppose each other, they work together to make us function properly. We need both parts to lead healthy lives. In fact every time you breathe in, your sympathetic nervous system is stimulated, and every time you exhale, your parasympathetic nervous system is stimulated. As you can imagine, both are being used hundreds of times each day, usually without you noticing anything. The figure below shows some of the many physiological functions controlled by these two halves of the autonomic nervous system.

Autonomic Nervous System

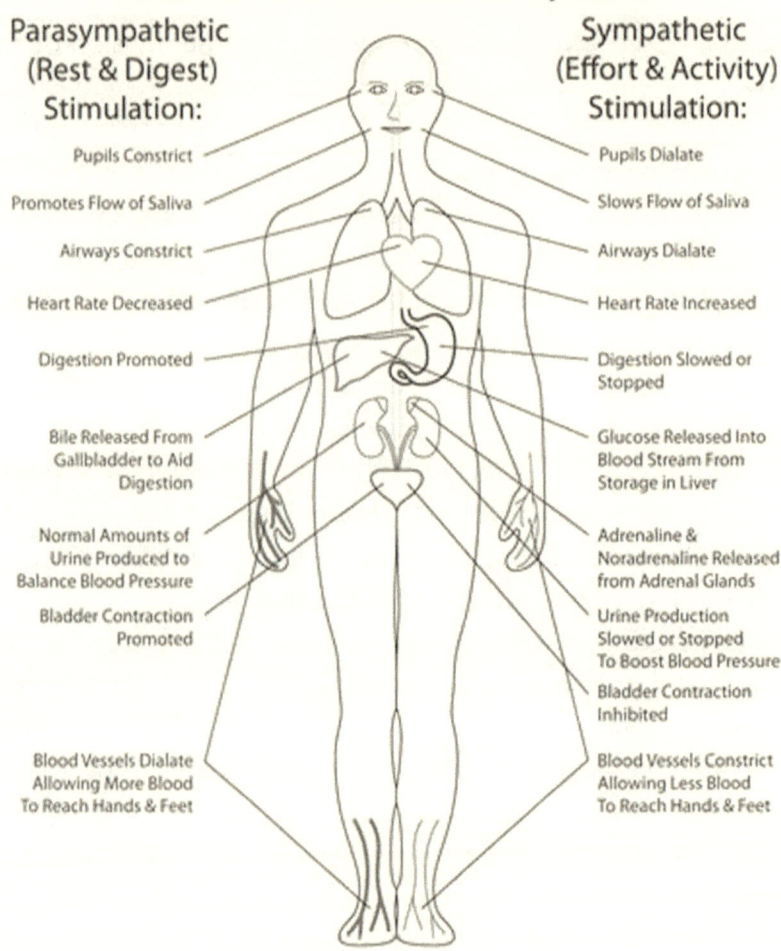

Parasympathetic (Rest & Digest) Stimulation:

- Pupils Constrict
- Promotes Flow of Saliva
- Airways Constrict
- Heart Rate Decreased
- Digestion Promoted
- Bile Released From Gallbladder to Aid Digestion
- Normal Amounts of Urine Produced to Balance Blood Pressure
- Bladder Contraction Promoted
- Blood Vessels Dialate Allowing More Blood To Reach Hands & Feet

Sympathetic (Effort & Activity) Stimulation:

- Pupils Dialate
- Slows Flow of Saliva
- Airways Dialate
- Heart Rate Increased
- Digestion Slowed or Stopped
- Glucose Released Into Blood Stream From Storage in Liver
- Adrenaline & Noradrenaline Released from Adrenal Glands
- Urine Production Slowed or Stopped To Boost Blood Pressure
- Bladder Contraction Inhibited
- Blood Vessels Constrict Allowing Less Blood To Reach Hands & Feet

PARASYMPATHETIC NERVOUS SYSTEM

As the diagram above illustrates, the parasympathetic nervous system controls many of the body's vital systems. It is often referred to as the *rest and digest* part of the nervous system because of its central role in promoting digestion and sleep. While this nickname is a good way to remember the function of the parasympathetic nervous system, it's a bit misleading. While sleep and digestion are two of the more conspicuous roles of the parasympathetic nervous system, it controls a lot more than that.

The parasympathetic nervous system, when stimulated, promotes healing and recovery throughout the body, strengthens the immune system, and controls dozens of other functions. The healing and recovery stimulated by the parasympathetic nervous system occur on a cellular level, making them hard to notice. However, these unseen processes are critically important for recovery from diseases that result from chronic stress. For that reason we like to refer to the parasympathetic nervous system as the *recovery and healing* part of the nervous system. (We know it doesn't rhyme, but it's a lot more meaningful.)

In addition to recovering from injury and disease, the *recovery and healing* part of the nervous system is needed on a daily basis. In fact it's essential for survival. Our bodies face constant wear and tear from the activities of life. This means that even healthy individuals must repair or replace damaged or dying cells throughout the body every day. This intensive process is vital to health, and it's the job of the parasympathetic nervous system to make sure it happens. For that reason a strong parasympathetic nervous system is important for anyone who wants to be healthy, and it's even more important for those suffering from chronic pain or disease.

THE SYMPATHETIC NERVOUS SYSTEM

The figure found at the end of the Involuntary Nervous System section shows that the sympathetic nervous system also controls many important functions throughout the body. It has its own nickname too, one you're probably much more familiar with—the fight-or-flight response. Once again, this nickname is a great way to remember the difference between the two parts of the involuntary nervous system, but it can be very misleading. The biggest misnomer that comes from this nickname is the idea that the sympathetic nervous system is only stimulated when you are in extreme danger or fear for your life. The truth is that the sympathetic nervous system is stimulated every time you stand up, go for a walk, or any other activity that requires effort. It is much better to think of the sympathetic nervous system as the *effort and activity* part of the involuntary nervous system. This more accurately describes its normal everyday role in the physiology of a healthy person.

How the Sympathetic and Parasympathetic Systems Interact

When one-half of the autonomic nervous system is stimulated, it stops (inhibits) the other *(Sapolsky 2004, 23)*. This means that when the sympathetic nervous system is stimulated, it prevents healing and recovery, in addition to all the other effects of the parasympathetic nervous system. Likewise, parasympathetic stimulation inhibits the sympathetic system. Both halves of the autonomic system are important for a healthy life, but they must be balanced. As you will learn later, an imbalance in frequency or strength of stimulation on either side can lead to serious consequences for your health.

While the sympathetic nervous system is important and necessary for a healthy, productive life, it is best to have your autonomic scale tilted toward the parasympathetic side. The sympathetic side is the bully of the two and must be kept in check. An overactive parasympathetic system is extremely rare, so you don't need to worry about that aspect.

It's also important to understand that neither side is an all-or-nothing affair. Both can be stimulated at various intensities. You can think of the nervous system as operating on a spectrum (see diagram below), with a totally relaxed vegetative state on one end and a crazed fight-or-flight response on the other end. Living at either extreme is not healthy; again the goal is balance. When referring to balance we mean that when you experience a peak in sympathetic stimulation, a peak in parasympathetic stimulation should eventually follow it, allowing you to recover from the excitement.

While the autonomic system is a spectrum, there is no absolute middle where neither side is stimulated. One side is always engaged. I'm sure you can guess which one should be your baseline. That's right, the good old *rest and recovery* side. For optimum health we should try to spend most of our time living with mild parasympathetic stimulation, just left of the middle of the spectrum diagram found following this section. We will always experience peaks in stimulation on both sides of the spectrum throughout the day. The key is to quickly return to a healthy baseline. The figure below will help you visualize these two parts of the involuntary nervous system.

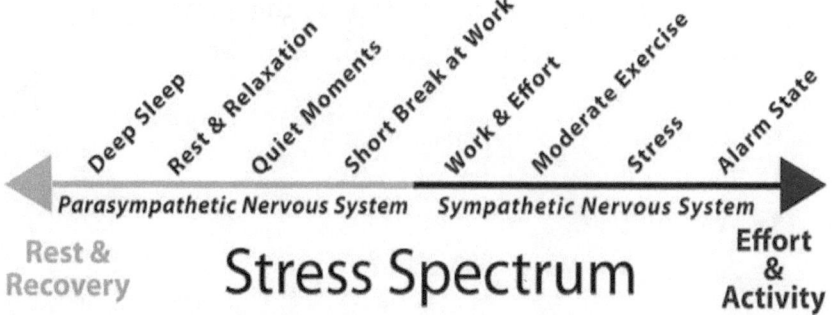

ALARM STATE (FIGHT OR FLIGHT)

Before moving on we want to describe some of the physiological changes that occur when the sympathetic nervous system is in full swing, the response often called *fight or flight*. Understanding the *fight-or-flight* response will help you understand why it's best to minimize sympathetic stimulation whenever possible. The importance of a strong parasympathetic response becomes most clear against a backdrop of constant sympathetic stimulation.

We've all experienced the *fight-or-flight response* at some point in our lives. Its effect on the body is widespread and quite remarkable in its ability to prepare us for life-threatening situations. When confronted with extreme danger, there are a host of changes that occur throughout the body without us consciously thinking about them. Some of these responses, and the problems they can lead to, are listed below.

- Increased heart rate
- Increased blood pressure
- Increased blood glucose
- Increased blood flow to large muscles in legs, torso, and arms
- Decreased blood flow to skin, internal organs, hands, and feet
- Fine motor skills (steady speech, writing, etc.) are sacrificed for gross motor skills (running, jumping, etc.).
- Pupils of the eye dilate to allow in more light to see clearly.
- Reaction time quickens.
- Digestion slows down or stops.
- And more...

These are really useful responses if you need to fight or run for your life. But, as you can imagine, these responses are not something you want to experience on a regular basis. In addition to the large-scale changes listed above, cellular healing and repair are also brought to a halt while your body marshals all resources toward the impending real or imagined danger.

While we doubt you are experiencing this level of intense sympathetic stimulation on a regular basis, there is a reason for explaining this "alarm state." All the changes that occur in your body when you are in extreme danger happen on a smaller scale any time your sympathetic nervous system is over stimulated or continuously stimulated. Many of those responses, even when mild, are harmful if they occur on a frequent or sustained basis. Even worse they often go unrecognized. The list below shows how many of the responses stimulated by the sympathetic nervous system become damaging if they continue for too long.

- Increased blood pressure→ chronic high blood pressure
- Increased blood glucose→ blood glucose dysregulation, diabetes, cardiovascular disease
- Decreased blood flow to skin, internal organs, hands, and feet→ decreased fuel supply to vital organs and extremities
- Pupils of the eye dilate to allow in more light to see clearly→ sensitivity to light
- Digestion slows down or stops→ digestive dysfunction, malabsorption, etc.
- Increased systemic inflammation→ widespread inflammatory responses throughout the body
- Just to name a few...

The bottom line is that frequent or sustained sympathetic stimulation is bad for everyone. As we mentioned earlier, it's best to spend most of your time slightly left of center on the stress spectrum above. This is not a simple task, especially since we may not realize we are on the *effort and activity* side of the spectrum or know what is putting us on that side of the spectrum in the first place.

THE STRESS RESPONSE

The *stress response* is a general name given to the group of physiological changes brought about by the sympathetic nervous system in response to *stressors*. To initiate those physiological changes, the sympathetic nervous system affects organ systems either directly through nerve signals or through the release of a special cocktail of stress hormones. The hormonal response to stress is quite complex and powerful and includes a few hormones you've probably heard of, including adrenaline (epinephrine), noradrenaline (norepinephrine), and a unique group of hormones called glucocorticoids (including cortisol) *(Sapolsky 2004, 22, 30; Chestnut 2005, 35-38; Karatsoreos and McEwen 2011, 581).*

The purpose of the stress response is to deal with *stressors* and to bring the body back into a balanced state. Humans, like most organisms, are constantly trying to stay in a balanced physiological state. For example, we are constantly regulating our body temperature to keep us from getting too hot or too cold. When we get too hot, sympathetic stimulation causes us to sweat, cooling us down. When we get too cold, sympathetic stimulation causes us to shiver, creating heat in the muscles and restricting blood flow to the arms and legs so our internal organs stay warm. Being too hot or too cold is considered a stressor, and the response the body takes to that stress is called the *stress response.* *The intention of the* **stress response** *is to bring the body back into a balanced state.* (This is referred to as homeostasis.) Interestingly, the *stress response* can be mild or intense depending on how the body interprets the severity of the stressor.

Due to our modern lifestyles, there are an endless number of stressors the body can encounter—some are physical, chemical, environmental, or neurological (like we briefly discussed), while others are psychological. However, the ways that the body attempts to rebalance itself from these stressors, whether mild or intense, is surprisingly consistent *(Sapolsky 2004, 10–11; Karatsoreos and McEwen 2011).*

For example, your body will respond to a public speaking engagement in much the same way as a nearly averted car accident. The measured sympathetic response is useful in the case of an averted car accident. It sharpens your focus and attention for the task at hand (regaining control of your car). For a public-speaking engagement, well you know how that goes. Your voice may become unsteady, and your hands shake. You can't think clearly, and you may start sweating profusely even in a chilly conference room. Obviously, this type of response to public speaking is neither necessary nor beneficial.

The similarity in our biological response to vastly different stressors doesn't necessarily make sense for our lives today, but it's the biology we are stuck with. The human body's generalized response to different stressors is likely due to our historical past. Our ancestors' answer to almost every problem was to either run or fight.

You don't need to remember all these details. The key concept is simple. The various responses our bodies go through in an attempt to rebalance themselves when faced with stressors is called the *stress response*. And, while certain small details change based on the type of stressor, many of the responses remain the same *(Sapolsky 2004, 10)*.

How Rebalancing Works with a Balanced Autonomic Nervous System

In those with a healthy, balanced autonomic system, the body's reaction to a stressor roughly follows the steps listed below.

1. The body is exposed to an internal or external stressor.

2. The brain responds to that stressor by stimulating the sympathetic nervous system.

3. Through various physiological changes, the sympathetic nervous system enables the body to resolve the stressor.

4. With the stressor eliminated, the body is brought back into balance. The sympathetic nervous system is no longer needed, and the parasympathetic nervous system is stimulated.

In reality, this process is more complex, but the general idea is what really matters to you. The *stress response* is supposed to be a short-term response that enables the body to deal with a stressor. Afterward, the body should quickly return to a normal, balanced state so you can move on with the rest of your life. This entire process is coordinated by the brain and occurs at varying degrees of intensity, dozens of times throughout the day.

This never-ending balancing act is part of having a healthy and balanced autonomic nervous system. Small, everyday stressors are quickly dealt with, and the body moves back into a balanced autonomic range. The following diagram shows how these spikes in the sympathetic nervous system (due to stress) occur throughout the day. Notice how the spikes in sympathetic stimulation are short lived then followed by a return to the balance zone. The result is a healthy autonomic system where peaks in *effort and activity* are balanced out with peaks in *recovery and healing.*

Balanced Autonomic System

(Neuro-Balance)

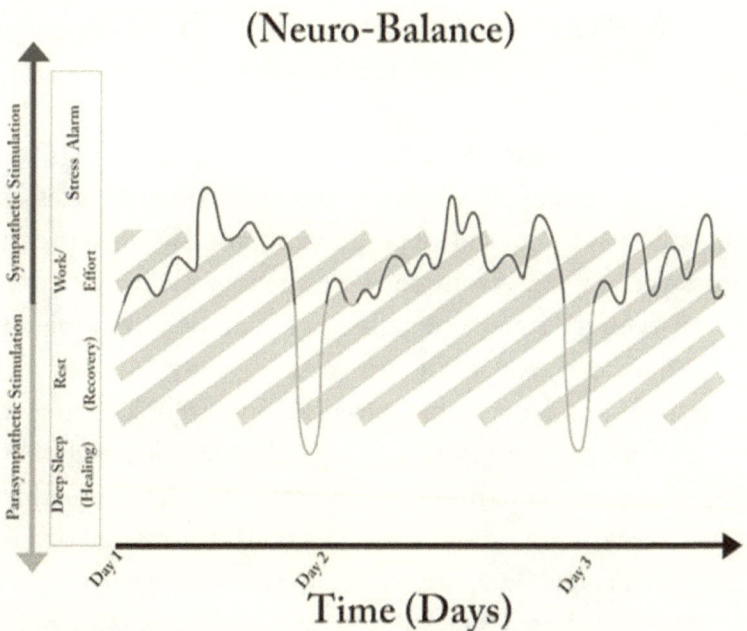

Time (Days)

As the diagram above illustrates, healthy individuals should spend most of their time near the center of the stress spectrum (inside the balance zone). Peaks in sympathetic stimulation (*effort and activity*) are quickly brought back into the balance zone by mild parasympathetic stimulation, allowing the body to rest and recover from stressors. This graph is a great way to understand the body's dynamic way of dealing with stressors. Although the autonomic system is in a constant state of flux, it can still be in balance. This dynamic balancing act, which the body is constantly experiencing, is called *allostasis (McEwen and Stellar 1993,*

2093–101). Allostasis describes the way the autonomic nervous system seeks balance in an ever-changing world. Just as in the previous chapters, for the sake of simplicity we will refer to allostasis as *Neuro-Balance.*

STRESS, STRESSORS, AND THREE TYPES OF STRESS RESPONSES

The concept of stress has taken on numerous meanings in the past several decades. We most commonly think of stress as a nonspecific psychological phenomenon, and the interpretation of stress varies widely from person to person. Because stress has taken on such a slippery meaning, we will avoid talking about stress and instead talk about stressors.

Stressors are identifiable physical or psychological events that elicit the *stress response* from our bodies. While psychological stressors can be more difficult to identify, they are indeed *stressors* that have real physiological effects on the body. For example, if you are nervous or upset, you can have gastrointestinal disturbances and altered digestion. The consequences of psychological stress can manifest themselves in the body in numerous concrete and measurable ways. Over the past several decades, this notion—which was once thought questionable—has become a respected scientific field known as *stress physiology.**

Psychological stress is an important topic, but this book is not specifically designed to help you deal with these kinds of stressors. For the most part, when we refer to stressors throughout this book, we're referring to physical stressors (either internal

---

* If you want to learn more about how psychological stress affects your physiology, we highly recommend reading Robert Sapolsky's book *Why Zebras Don't Get Ulcers.* It's a witty and entertaining read that is highly informative.

or environmental) that affect the body. Environmental stressors are often categorized as either acute or silent.

Acute stressors—These are obvious threats to our survival, things like violent encounters, life-threatening danger, major wounds, and serious infections.

Silent stressors—These stressors can come from many different sources, including our diet, toxins, parasitic infections, low-grade bacterial infections, silent inflammation, lack of sleep, temperature extremes, lack of food, excessive visual stimulation from television, video games, cell phones, and the list goes on. Silent stressors can be quite insidious because we are usually unaware of them. Many times they don't cause obvious symptoms. After all, if we were aware of these stressors, we would probably stop exposing ourselves to them or seek professional treatment. For that reason we refer to these low-level stressors as *silent stress.*

There are certain types of stressors that the body can handle while still maintaining its dynamic autonomic balance. Aside from the constant mild stressors we go through, like getting out of a chair or going for a walk, people with balanced autonomic nervous systems are quite adept at handling infrequent acute stressors.

ACUTE STRESS RESPONSE (SHORT TERM)

Acute stressors elicit the type of *stress response* our brains and bodies are best equipped to deal with *(Moore 2011, Seaward 2011, Chestnut 2005, Sapolsky 2004, 4).* For example, a child darting in front of your car is an acute stressor. The sympathetic system is stimulated the moment you see the quickly moving child in your peripheral vision. The stress response immediately heightens your senses, quickens your heart rate, and improves your reaction times. It enables you to slam on the brakes quickly enough to avoid hitting the child. The stressor was dealt with, and sympathetic stimulation stops. Your hands may be shaky for a few minutes afterward, but, in most cases, your body is back to its normal baseline in a matter of minutes. The danger came and went; you dealt with it and are ready to move on. We can thank this type of stress response for saving us from countless catastrophes every year of our lives.

In fact acute stress actually helps to keep our brain active and healthy. This type of stress helps to maintain Neuromechanical Balance by challenging the brain's autonomic nervous system response (sympathetic) and recovery (parasympathetic). The key here is that there must be ample time between stressors to allow for recovery.

You now know how the body responds to "healthy" acute stressors. Hopefully this information allows you to see how a balanced autonomic system should function. Aside from the acute stress response, there are two other types of stress responses that eventually lead to *Neuro-Imbalance* (also known as *dysautonomia*).

FREQUENT-STRESS RESPONSE

The frequent-stress response is common in soldiers and emergency responders like law-enforcement officers, ambulance drivers, ER nurses, doctors, and fire fighters; however, it can also be seen in people with other high-stress jobs and lifestyles. This type of stress is best described as frequent false alarms. For example, when police are called to a crime scene or emergency, they have to be ready for anything. This means their sympathetic nervous system must be ramped up, so they can respond to an acute stressor at a moment's notice. The frequent-stress response is certainly not healthy, but a small number of people can handle this kind of stress fairly well *(Sapolsky 2004, 4)*.

The best example of those who effectively cope with the *frequent-stress response* is elite soldiers like the US Navy SEALs. Through extensive training and practice, elite soldiers have been conditioned to quickly elevate their sympathetic *fight-or-flight* response, while maintaining their ability to drop back into a relaxed parasympathetic state, so they can quickly recover from stress *(Taylor 2007, B224–30)*.

It is crucial to understand that these individuals are not successful simply because they can get pumped up quickly; most people can do that just fine. Their ability to quickly relax and recover after a stressful event is crucial to their success. In fact studies have shown that individuals who do not make the cut in elite special forces groups are those who have great difficulty stimulating their parasympathetic nervous system after stressful training events. These individuals suffer from burnout because their bodies are not able to rest and heal fast enough. In essence they aren't able to adequately rebalance their autonomic nervous system, resulting in an overstimulated sympathetic nervous system.

What does this have to do with you?

Well, if you aren't one of the lucky few who have a natural ability to cope with frequent stress events, having your sympathetic nervous system ramped up frequently will likely take a toll on your body. You may have great difficulty relaxing, preventing you from getting onto the recovery and healing side of the stress spectrum. You may get stuck in effort and activity mode with disastrous consequences for your health. We'll learn more about how and why this happens later on.

Keep in mind that the frequent-stress response isn't limited to those with dangerous occupations. Being repeatedly exposed to environmental stressors such as toxic mold, pesticides, polluted air, and poor sleep can cause the frequent-stress response too. However, if you have, or have had, one of the occupations listed above, you may be suffering from the frequent-stress response. The good news is this type of stress is often easier to address than the low-grade chronic stress discussed next, although the treatment strategies are the same.

LOW-GRADE CHRONIC STRESS RESPONSE

Any stressor you are exposed to on a more-or-less continuous basis can cause low-grade chronic stress. These stressors are often something you don't identify as stressful or harmful (silent stressors). In other words you don't realize these things are causing any health problems.

Often times there are multiple *silent stressors* contributing to low-grade chronic stress. These stressors can happen simultaneously, or you can move from exposure to one stressor to another throughout the week, month, or year. Below is a list of some common silent stressors that lead to low-grade chronic stress.

- High-inflammation diet
- Chronic sitting
- Lack of adequate deep sleep
- Shallow breathing
- Poor posture
- Continuous noise from a busy street by your home or office (noise pollution)
- Air pollution
- Chronic, low-grade infections

- Food sensitivities
- Environmental toxins (pesticides, herbicides, household cleaners, and fertilizers)
- Subclinical blood glucose dysregulation (dysglycemia)
- Poorly managed diabetes

Low-grade chronic stress can also come from psychological stressors like daily anxiety over your occupation, strained family relationships, or daily frustration with traffic on the way to work.

As you can see, low-grade chronic stress can originate from a wide number of sources. Due to its repetitive nature, this type of stress has both neurological and physiological consequences that not only damage the body but also have the ability to perpetuate the *stress response*.

We'll get into the detailed consequences of low-grade chronic stress a little later.

In the meantime the following consequences of silent stress should convince you to pay attention to low-grade chronic stress because of its role in many diseases.

- Arthritis—This is a result of uneven loading and inflammation in the joints (i.e. spinal decay) *(Scully 2010)*.
- Glucose dysregulation—This is bad for anyone but especially diabetics. This condition negatively affects the delivery of fuel to the brain and nerves *(Timmins 2011, 52; Sapolsky 2004, 60–61, 66; McKwen and Stellar 1993, 2093-2101)*.
- A suppressed immune system—This increases your chances of contracting bacterial and viral infections *(Timmins 2011, 53–4; Sapolsky 2004, 151–5; Chestnut 2005, 35-38, 43-55)*.

- Constriction of peripheral blood vessels in nonessential areas of the body and especially in the skin—This affects fuel delivery to the hands and feet *(Chestnut 2005, 28; Sapolsky 2004, 38)*.
- Decreased ability to repair and rebuild damaged tissues—This includes damaged discs *(Karlamangla et al. 2002, 696-710; Sapolsky 2004, 11; Chestnut 2005, 32)*.
- Accelerated aging of the brain—Effects of this include poor memory *(McEwen 2002, 921-936; Sapolsky 1996, 1–19; Chestnut 2005, 41-42)*.

The next diagram shows how both frequent and chronic stress responses affect the balance of the autonomic nervous system.

Imbalanced Autonomic System

(Neuro-Imbalance)

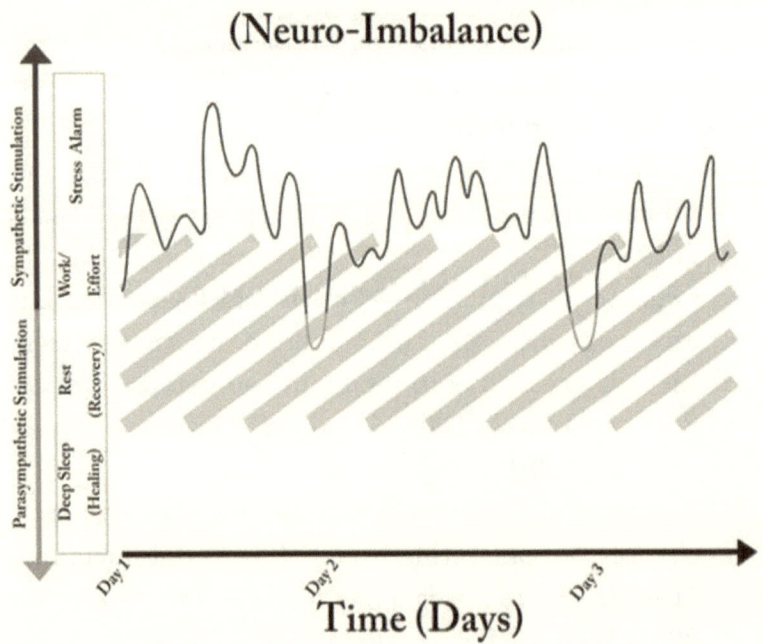

Do you notice how the peaks and troughs of autonomic stimulation have shifted upward into the *effort and activity* side of the spectrum? This means that autonomic balance is lost. Sympathetic stimulation spikes and drops, but the low points are either still outside the healthy balance zone of the spectrum or only slightly into the parasympathetic side. A new baseline of sympathetic overstimulation is created.

Constant sympathetic overstimulation replaces the natural and healthy baseline of a balanced nervous system. This type of neurological imbalance causes a multitude of physical problems, and, over time, it is a major contributor to chronic diseases *(Sapolsky 2004, 6; Chestnut 2005, 54-55; McEwen et al. 2012; Karlamangla et al. 2002, 696-710).* Neurological imbalance, in our clinical experience, is frequently the missing link in the effective management of chronic conditions.

Understanding how and why neurological imbalance contributes to your stress levels is the key to successful management of your pain, and that is the focus of the next section *(McEwen 2002, 921-936; Moore et al. 2011, 20; Ludke and Rothe 2014, 6).*

CHAPTER 14

THE CHRONIC STRESS CYCLE

KEY POINTS

- *The chronic stress cycle* occurs when autonomic imbalance goes on for too long, and you are stuck in chronic stress response.
- Due to the brain being very efficient, an ongoing neuro-imbalance will allow your brain to adapt and actually become very good at being imbalanced. Thus, an ongoing neuro-imbalance will create chronic stress, which will perpetuate the imbalance.
- Because Neuro-Imbalance is "silent," it requires special forms of testing to be assessed. *The gold standard in testing for Neuro-Imbalance is heart-rate variability.*
- Neuro-Imbalance commonly leads to many problems: mechanical imbalances, blood-sugar problems, poor sleep, digestive problems, whole-body inflammation, immune-system problems, autoimmune diseases, adrenal problems, brain disorders, as well as heart and vascular disease.

If you recall from earlier, the dynamic autonomic balancing act that occurs in healthy individuals is simply called *Neuro-Balance*. When the autonomic system becomes unbalanced, and its baseline shifts into the sympathetic side of the stress spectrum, a damaging phenomenon called *Neuro-Imbalance* occurs. When the Neuro-Imbalance is not addressed, an even more damaging process called the chronic stress cycle can occur.

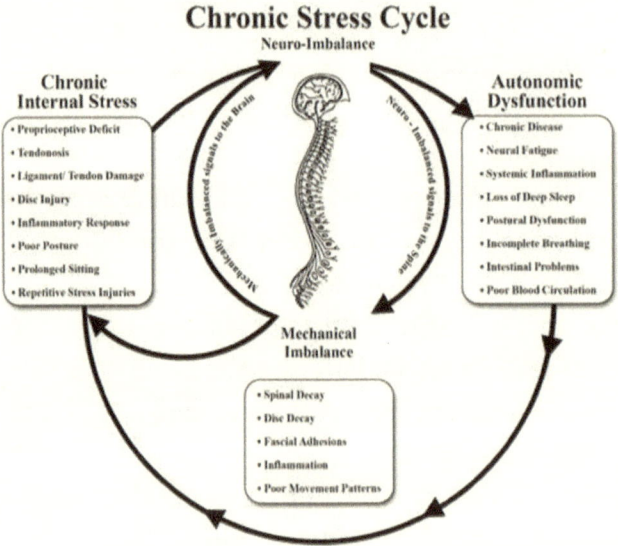

This process can be initiated by frequent-stress response or by chronic, low-level stress response. The original stressors stimulate the sympathetic nervous system in the brain, resulting in the stress response. Unlike the healthy stress response where an acute stressor is quickly dealt with and resolved, frequent or chronic stressors cause the brain to produce a persistent stress response.

During a healthy stress response, the physiological changes the body makes are healthy and adaptive. They enable us to more effectively deal with the stressor at hand. When stressors are frequent or chronic those same adaptive responses become unhealthy and maladaptive. Maladaptive responses reduce our ability to deal with stress and reduce our overall level of health through a process called Neuro-Imbalance.

Neuro-imbalance is a complex idea, but the basics are pretty simple. Because the stress response is a short-sighted process with the goal of survival, it squanders large amounts of energy and resources. Many of the physiological changes that occur under sympathetic stimulation are costly and inefficient, and the byproducts of those changes can be damaging in the long run. In addition the cocktail of stress hormones released during the stress response is meant for short-term use only; when these hormones are present in the blood stream for too long or too often, they cause serious problems. Neuro-Imbalance describes the physical cost of dealing with an overactive stress response including the strain on the body's energy and nutrient resources *(McEwen and Stellar 1993, 2093–101)*. If you live with Neuro-Imbalance long enough, it will lead to wear and tear on the body.

TESTING FOR NEURO-IMBALANCE

Although heart-rate variability is the gold standard, there are a number of biomarkers (blood, urine, or saliva test parameters) that are highly correlated with autonomic imbalance *(Sztajzel 2004, 514–22)*. If a blood test reveals that several of these markers are above the functional rage, it is very likely you are suffering from Neuro-Imbalance. Below is a list of the common lab test markers associated with autonomic imbalance *(Glei et al. 2007, 769–76; Ludke and Rothe 2014, 6-7; Gruenewald et al. 2006, 14158-14163)*.

- Glycosylated hemoglobin, fasting glucose
- Cholesterol measurements
- C-reactive protein
- Salivary Cortisol
- DHEAs
- Lymphocytes, natural killer cells, macrophages
- Albumin
- Fibrinogen
- Homocysteine

DAMAGE CAUSED BY NEURO-IMBALANCE

The wear and tear *Neuro-Imbalance* causes eventually accumulates, resulting in damage and dysfunction in various systems throughout the body. The exact type of damage and dysfunction that result depend on your health history and genetics. Here is a list of common effects of Neuro-Imbalance that lead to the chronic stress cycle.

- **Glucose dysregulation (prediabetes/diabetes)**— The stress response causes your body to boost the amount of glucose in the blood stream and dampen the effect of the hormone insulin (whose job it is to remove glucose from the blood stream) (Sapolsky 2004, 60; Karatsoreos and McEwen 2011, 581). When stress peaks repeatedly throughout the day, glucose shifts back and forth from its storage places in the body. The end result is chronically high blood glucose, because your body is busy preparing you for vigorous physical activity that never happens. In the short term, this is not a problem. When this process happens for too long, it contributes to Neuro-Imbalance. Here's why.

First, shifting glucose to and from its storage places throughout the body is energy intensive. When this process is done repeatedly, it can lead to chronic fatigue syndrome or a general lack of energy and vitality *(Sapolsky 2004, 62)*. Second, the energy resources that are diverted for this back-and-forth shift of glucose cannot be used to repair damaged tissues in your body. When damaged cells aren't fully repaired, they deteriorate. This is a double whammy for nerves because the excess glucose damages them, and the lack of energy to repair damaged tissues prevents those very same damaged nerves from recovering. In addition when this stress-induced glucose dysregulation occurs in those who already have high blood glucose or insulin resistance, it can lead to diabetes.

- **Silent Inflammation**—Neuro-Imbalance, acting as a stressor, promotes the release of stress hormones by the sympathetic nervous system. Glucocorticoids, an important class of hormones associated with stress, reduce inflammation in the body. However, long-term exposure to high levels of glucocorticoids can blunt the effect of these important inflammation-reducing hormones *(Cohen et al. 2012, 5995–9; Bosmaden Boer and van Wetten and Pruimboom 2012, 32)*. The end result is a condition where the body has difficulty regulating inflammation, resulting in excessive inflammatory responses throughout the body. This is a major source of additional damage and dysfunction since most chronic diseases are inflammatory.

- **Digestive Dysfunction and Malabsorption**—Hormones released during the stress response cause digestion to slow way down *(Williams et al. 1987, G582–6)*. Less acid is secreted in the stomach; fewer digestive enzymes are released into the small intestines. And there are fewer contractions of the small intestines, which move food through your diges-tive tract *(Thompson and Richelson and Malagelada 1983, 277–83)*.

The end result is a gastrointestinal nightmare. Now you'll be more likely to have all sorts of digestive upsets includ-ing inflammation caused by food that begins rotting in your intestines. This occurs when bacteria, fungus, and parasites survive the trip through your stomach due to lower-than-normal levels of stomach acid and slower movement of food through the small intestines *(Bures et al. 2010, 2978–90)*. You also won't be properly breaking apart (digesting) your food, which prevents your body from getting the vitamins and nutrients you need to stay healthy. The nasty side effects don't stop there; eventually they can lead to irritable bowel syndrome and put you at high risk of developing inflammatory bowel disease.

In fact digestion and malabsorption can lead to Neuro-Imbalance. But how does this happen? Your body ends up spending a lot of energy and nutrients fighting off excess bacte-ria in the intestines. Meanwhile the sad shape of your intestines prevents needed nutrients from being absorbed from your food. You can see how this creates a vicious cycle. Once again the net result is less energy to put into repairing damaged tissues and possible vitamin deficiencies.

- **Intestinal Permeability**—Intestinal permeability simply means that the body is allowing things to enter the blood stream when it shouldn't. The intes-tines act like a gatekeeper allowing only water and nutrients from the fully broken down food particles into the blood. When the gatekeeper is no longer working effectively, then too many particles will travel through the intestinal lining and into the blood when they shouldn't.

Long-term exposure to both physical and psychological stress increases intestinal permeability. This has been demonstrated in numerous studies on animals *(Söderholm and Perdue 2001, G7–G13; M Zareie et al. 2006, 1553–1560)*. Increased intestinal permeability can, in turn, lead to a number of additional health problems and stressors including autoimmune disorders, food sensitivities and allergies, silent inflammation, and others.

- **Immune System Dysfunction (including auto-immune diseases)**—The stress response suppresses immune function. More specifically, several of the hormones released in the stress response suppress immune function. They do so in several ways. These hormones reduce the production of various immune cells, remove some of these immune cells from circulation in the body, and—in the case of extreme stressors—can actually destroy them *(McEwen 1998, 171-179; Sapolsky 2004, 151–2)*.

As counterintuitive as it may seem given the explanation above, an overactive stress response is also closely linked to autoimmune diseases. While the exact reasons are not yet known, numerous studies have shown that there is a link between stress and autoimmunity *(Karlamangla et al 2002; Singer, B., Ryff, C. D., & Seeman 2004; Sapolsky 2004, 158–9)*.

- **Adrenal Dysfunction**—The stress response relies heavily on a few stress hormones produced in the adrenal glands to get you ready for action. The trouble is that stress hormones can block or suppress many other hormones, which help us function properly and feel good. As you probably guessed, this "stress hormone take-over" is good in the short term (if your life is threatened), but in the long run, it spells disaster for your health. In addition to blocking and suppressing many hormones, the stress hormones are made from the same building block as other important hormones. In the end, stress hormones not only block and suppress normal healthy hormones; they also prevent more healthy hormones from being made *(Timmins 2011, 48; McEwen 1998)*.

As long as your brain is telling you that you're stressed out, it will continue telling the organs in the body that produce hormones to keep pumping out the wrong ones. At the end of the day, this hormonal imbalance is the root of many of the other problems described below, since these stress hormones orchestrate much of the stress response *(Seaward 2011, 38-39; McEwen 1998, 171-179; Sapolsky 2004, 30–32)*.

- **Neurological Dysfunction**—Over time some of the hormones released during the stress response will damage an area of the brain called the hippocampus. This can result in learning difficulties and poor memory, as well as a variety of other neurological problems, including accelerated aging of the brain and even dementia *(Ferrari et al. 2001, 319–29; Karlamangla et. al. 2002, 696-710; Sapolsky 2004, 220)*.

- **Stress-Response-Induced Sleep Disruption**—The stress response releases hormones that suppress sleep *(Vgontzas and Chrousos 2002, 15–36)*. A lack of sleep, or poor sleep quality, further stimulates the stress response, potentially leading to chronic fatigue

(Sapolsky 2004, 237). Why is that so bad? Well, as you know from earlier, the stress response reduces the body's ability to repair and maintain damaged tissues. Put simply, without sleep we have a really hard time healing damaged cells. Over time lack of good sleep adds to your Neuro-Imbalance, causing wear and tear on your body *(McEwen 2006, S20–3).*

- **Hemisphericity**—Recent studies suggest that there is a link between stressful events and a lateralization of brain function. Stressors are able to cause an imbalance in brain function between the two lobes of the brain. This imbalance, known as lateralization or hemisphericity, can itself elicit a stress response by stimulating the production of stress hormones *(Braun 2007, 397-427; Karatsoreos and McEwen 2011, 579-582; Bob 2008, 185–91).* So a stressful event can cause hemisphericity, which in turn can cause a chronic stress response. This continual stimulation of the stress response leads to an amplified Neuro-Imbalance.

- **Cardiovascular Disease**—The stress response causes an increase in heart rate and blood pressure. When this continues for an extended period of time, this adaptive response takes a toll on the body. It causes increased wear and tear on your cardiovascular system damaging arteries, vessels, and capillaries and eventually causing them to become inflamed, which is the basis of cardiovascular disease. This inflammation depletes your body's energy and reduces its ability to deliver oxygen and nutrients to the brain. The nerves, which are especially sensitive to changes in oxygen and glucose, are damaged in the process.

The types of damage and dysfunction listed above can contribute to your back pain. But the damage doesn't stop there; these problems can also serve as additional stressors, which turn the normal self-terminating stress response into a dangerous self-perpetuating cycle. With more stressors feeding into the system, the stress response becomes more intense, leading to greater neurological imbalance. The increased wear and tear on the body intensifies the damage and dysfunction that is already under way. This is the *chronic stress cycle*. It's an extremely dangerous process that occurs at some level in most of the US population. Once it begins, targeted therapies are needed to slow or stop the damage that's underway.

If you have Neuro-Imbalance long enough, the chronic stress cycle can become self-perpetuating. The cycle is no longer dependent on external stressors.

Let us explain...

The self-perpetuating chronic stress cycle starts when the brain "rewires" itself for a sustained stress response. This rewiring occurs due to a phenomenon called neuroplasticity. Neurologists often explain this concept with the phrase *neurons that fire together wire together.* To understand what this means, we're going to give you a crash course on how the brain works.

Our brains are full of nerve cells called neurons, which connect to and communicate with other neurons around them. This communication is sometimes referred to as *firing.* It's kind of like a chain reaction where one neuron is stimulated, which in turn stimulates the neurons it connects to. The end result of these chain reactions may be a thought, a movement, or stimulation of the sympathetic nervous system. These chain reactions occur in different parts of the brain all the time; that's how the brain works. The more often a certain pattern or sequence of neurons is fired to produce the desired response, the better the brain gets at doing that task. This improvement occurs when the neurons involved develop a more efficient network of connections. In essence neurons that are frequently fired together become better connected or wired together—hence the phrase *neurons that fire together wire together (Doidge 2007; Pascual-Leone et al. 2005, 377–401; Pascual-Leone et al. 2001, 302–15).*

What does this have to do with the stress response? The stress response is just another pattern of firing neurons in the brain. In this case the desired effect is the stimulation of the sympathetic nervous system and the release of stress hormones. The more often you engage the stress response and fire that pattern, the more efficient the stress response becomes. The neurons involved become wired together quite well. If the group of neurons creating the stress response fire together often enough, that pattern can turn into a bad neurological habit.

Perhaps equally important, the neurons that regulate and stop the stress response actually shrink and become less connected when exposed to stress hormones over long periods of time. Lastly, neurons that normally regulate our response to potentially stressful events begin to shrink and become less interconnected during long periods of stress. The net result is a brain that has learned to be both hypersensitive to stress and a brain with a weakened ability to stop the stress response once it is initiated *(McEwen and Gianaros 2011, 431–45).*

Whew...you now know more about neurology than you probably ever cared to. Hopefully you see the importance of this concept of neuroplasticity. The brain optimizes itself based on what it does most frequently. This is how we master new skills and create new habits, good and bad.

When the stress response is frequently or constantly stimulated, the brain literally becomes hardwired for the stress response. The result is an autonomic system that is way out of balance. The brain may continue to initiate or perpetuate a stress response without any outside stimulus. This is called the (self-perpetuating) chronic stress cycle, which magnifies and reinforces Neuro-Imbalance, leading to Neuromechanical Imbalance as well as silent inflammation, chronic disease, and wear and tear throughout the body.

"In-Office" Testing

Earlier in this book, we described some of the testing we typically use for Neuro-Imbalances. A more detailed explanation of our in office tests is listed below.

- **Pulse Oximetry and O$_2$ Perfusion Test**—This test measures sympathetic stimulation by looking at blood circulation and oxygen concentration in the hands and feet *(Vegfors et al. 1990, 1–4; Yamazaki and Nishiyama and Suzuki 2012, 9–14).*

- **Heart Rate Variability (HRV)**—A patient's overall autonomic balance can be determined by looking at small natural variation in heart rate. Heart rate variability testing is the gold standard for identifying sympathetic overstimulation *(Goldman 2007; Grunewald et al. 2006; Sztajzel 2004, 514–22).*

- **SEMG (surface electromyography)**—This is a noninvasive test to check and compare the activity of the superficial muscles from side to side. The side of sympathetic dominance will be indicated on a graph that will show the need to balance the system. The goal is to have both sides fairly equal and within normal ranges of activity.

- **Salivary Cortisol Tests**—These tests measure the amount of cortisol that is being released in your body at any given time. The measurements are calculated through saliva collections over a specified number of hours throughout the course of a set number of days. Cortisol is the hormone released to wake you up in the morning, to break your fast throughout the night, and to prepare for a day's work. It is also released to mobilize your body's energy stores when you want to engage in activity. However, cortisol becomes unregulated and is released in high amounts when a person's sympathetic nervous system is in overdrive.
- **Function Neurological Tests**—These are completely non-invasive tests done with the help of electronics or by a clinician's trained eye. Trained doctors may check any combination of reflexes, specified eye movements and features, posturing, muscle tone, skin features, movement patterns, etc. to be able to determine the areas of lower function or, in this case, too much function. The tests are used pre- and post-treatment to determine the best direction for care.

CHAPTER 15

REDUCING NEURO-IMBALANCE

KEY POINTS

- Due to the complex nature of low back pain and chronic stress, changes in lifestyle are necessary to counteract the chronic stressors of everyday life.
- *If you* are *eager to begin restoring balance and do not yet have access to a doctor who can help you, the DICE protocol is an excellent place to start.*

By this point you fully understand the importance of maintaining a balanced autonomic system. This means spending as much time as possible on the *healing and recovery* side of the stress spectrum or, at the very least, moving closer to the center of the stress spectrum. Making that happen is the key to successful management of low back pain and other chronic conditions.

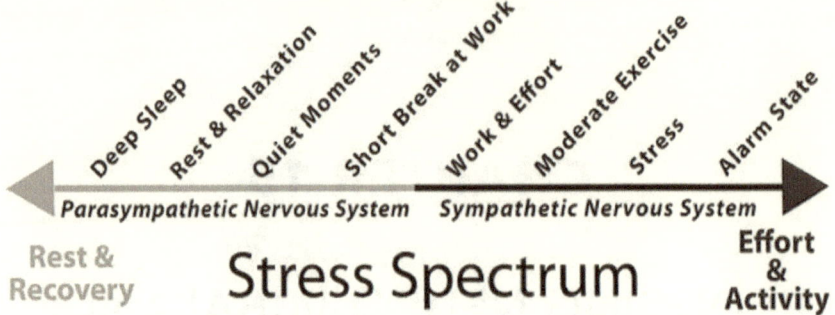

The major focuses required to break the chronic stress cycle include the following.

- Healing the damaged passive structures of the spine—The consequences of mechanical imbalance, such as spinal decay and disc degeneration, are themselves stressors that add to the chronic stress response.

- Reducing the Neuromechanical Imbalance that is also a stressor and adds to the chronic stress cycle—By restoring Neuromechanical Balance, we, in turn, are able to significantly reduce the Neuro-Imbalance (autonomic imbalance) resulting in system-wide healing effects throughout the body.

- Lifestyle changes—These changes reduce the avoidable stressors that, in turn, trigger the chronic stress cycle. (This is the DICE protocol.)

The first two areas of focus mentioned above are, of course, our two-part approach for treating back pain. However, there is a third (and very important) part to our two-part approach that is necessary to break the chronic stress cycle, stop your back pain, and improve all aspects of your life.

We know it doesn't make sense to have a third part of a two-part approach, but since we wrote the book, we can take liberties in logic. In reality the two-part approach includes the interventions that we do in our office, and the third part includes lifestyle changes, not clinical interventions.

Part three of this book is a detailed how-to guide for each of the strategies that make up the DICE protocol. Incorporating these lifestyle strategies under the guidance of a qualified health-care professional will enable you to reduce your chronic stress, often significantly.

REDUCING CHRONIC STRESSORS

It is impossible to completely eliminate chronic stress in our lives. We live in a constantly changing world where external stressors are all around us, and the ever-present internal stressors cannot be avoided. These unavoidable stressors will always create some level of Neuro-Imbalance. What's great is that you don't have to completely eliminate this imbalance to manage your condition. Instead, the DICE protocol provides you with concrete ways to reduce chronic stressors in your life. You can accomplish this by eliminating avoidable stressors when possible and learning to reduce and manage the unavoidable ones.

Using this realistic approach, most patients are able to reduce their chronic stress to a healthy and manageable level. This strategy allows them to more successfully manage their condition and, most importantly, their lives.

For this reduction to occur, we recommend a combination of simple, easy-to-follow strategies which can be done with little to no cost. We call these four lifestyle strategies the DICE protocol. You may remember that DICE stands for *Deep sleep, In-line posture, Complete breathing* and *Energy restoration diet.* The at-home strategies discussed in the following chapters of this book are recommended for nearly everyone; it's the closest thing to a cookie-cutter approach we could create. However, it is important for you to consult your doctor or health-care professional before starting any at-home therapy.

Part three of this book includes the breakdown of the DICE protocol and explains how you can begin reducing your chronic stress today.

PART III

STRATEGIES FOR REDUCING
CHRONIC STRESS
AT HOME AND WORK

CHAPTER 16

DICE PROTOCOL

The DICE protocol is not just for those suffering from back pain. These lifestyle strategies are universally helpful for anyone who wants to dramatically improve health, energy level, and sense of wellbeing. It's a simple program that can, by itself, dramatically improve your life. As you know from the previous chapter, the DICE protocol is aimed at lowering chronic stress, a major contributing factor to nearly all chronic health issues. For that reason reducing chronic stress is a powerful way to improve your general health and well-being.

Most people come into our office because of their pain, but they find that their lives are improved in ways they didn't think were possible. Simply put, reducing chronic stress using the DICE protocol makes you feel better!

As mentioned before DICE stands for Deep sleep, In-line posture, Complete breathing, and Energy-restoration diet. This section is divided into individual chapters describing each of these therapies. In these sections you'll not only learn simple strategies and lifestyle changes that will reduce your chronic stress, you'll also learn why these strategies work as well as some of the research behind them.

You may be wondering why exercise is not included in the DICE protocol. The truth is, it should be. However, when it comes to working with people in pain and those with low energy, exercise is simply not a realistic option (regardless of how effective it may be). The DICE protocol, along with the other strategies in this book, aims at reducing pain and boosting energy to the point that exercise becomes a realistic option. Once this happens, or if a person is already able to exercise, we highly recommend following the exercise strategies covered later in the book. Exercise truly is an essential factor to health, but it is oftentimes not a realistic part of early treatment.

Additionally, we've noticed that once patients start feeling better, they have a natural desire to boost their activity level and begin exercising more on their own. This is only natural since exercise makes us feel good, and for many people the pain is what causes them to stop exercising. Instead of the "exercise to feel good" mantra that we often hear from all the health experts, we have found that the "feel good to exercise" philosophy is much more successful in accomplishing long-term changes in patients with chronic health issues.

Many of these therapies are simple exercises or lifestyle changes that can be done with or without a doctor's direct oversight. This is good news if you are unable to see a doctor in your area who uses progressive non-drug therapies to treat back pain. However, you will still need to check with your doctor to make sure this program is right for you.

All the strategies and exercises in the following chapters are safe for the vast majority of low back pain sufferers. However, there may be some exercises that cause certain people pain due to special health conditions or past injuries. If you discover that an exercise causes pain, stop doing that exercise. If the pain doesn't go away, please consult your doctor. You should not experience pain or any other complications during any of the exercises in this program.

CHAPTER 17

DEEP SLEEP

Getting adequate sleep is a serious problem for countless Americans. And it's not just about feeling rested. A lack of quality sleep is a major factor in many chronic illnesses because of its importance in the healing process and in its contribution to maintaining balance within the autonomic nervous system. Because of the tendency for back-pain symptoms to worsen at the end of the day, getting adequate sleep can be a serious challenge. For those suffering from any condition, broken sleep is a difficult hurdle in a patient's path to healing.

If your pain is causing you to lose sleep, you are not alone. Many of our patients tell us they can learn to deal with the pain and discomfort of their sciatica or back pain during the day, but the restless nights and chronic lack of sleep puts them over the edge and seriously lowers their quality of life. How do you know if you are not getting adequate sleep? The simplest way is to track how many hours you sleep each night. Most adults need somewhere between seven and nine hours of sleep each night in order to feel their best, but hours alone don't give you the full picture. Your sleep quality can suffer while your total hours of sleep stay the same. This is a big problem.

As you may recall, inadequate sleep and poor-quality sleep are both stressors that contribute to the chronic stress cycle. For that reason a chronic lack of sleep and poor-quality sleep can be both a contributing factor and a symptom of spinal decay. It's another vicious cycle associated with pain. The simple fact is that, without adequate sleep, healing from any condition is very difficult. Yet for many getting adequate sleep is nearly impossible without some relief in their symptoms.

If your back symptoms are keeping you up at night, know this; getting a full night's sleep (including deep sleep) *is* possible. Getting a full night's sleep is one of the biggest milestones for our patients. It's not uncommon to have a patient confide in us that, for the first time in years, they are falling asleep more quickly and sleeping through the entire night. Getting better sleep is one of the many positive side effects of reducing the stress response and restoring the disc. But better sleep is not just a side effect; getting better sleep is also a crucial part of the program, one that helps reduce your chronic stress and gives your body a chance to heal.

Although the other strategies in the DICE protocol, as well as those discussed in later chapters, should enable you to sleep more easily, in and of themselves, there are a number of things you can do to start improving the quality of your sleep right away.

Before we get into those sleep strategies, you need to understand why adequate sleep—especially deep sleep—is so important to your health and how a constantly elevated stress response prevents restful sleep.

SLEEP AND HEALTH

Sleep is not only essential to heal from a sickness, it's also essential for maintaining your current level of health as well. Our human body is in a constant state of repair. Old cells eventually become tired and worn out and need to be replaced by new ones. The cells and tissues that are damaged throughout each day must be repaired or replaced if you want to stay healthy. If too many cells are damaged, and not repaired or replaced, your health will decline over time.

Much of the daily healing and repair work that occurs in the body occurs during nighttime sleep. Even more importantly the most intensive repair work occurs during a phase of sleep called *slow-wave sleep* or deep sleep. In fact studies have shown that there is a large pulse in the release of growth hormone (GH) during deep sleep *(Brandenberger and Weibel 2004, 251–5)*. Half of the total amount of growth hormone released through the day comes in this nighttime pulse, but this large pulse only occurs in those who experience adequate slow-wave sleep.

This is important because growth hormone has an indispensable role in stimulating the daily growth and repair of damaged cells throughout the body. For that reason experiencing this pulse in GH has widespread consequences for your health. The important point here is that it's not simply the duration of sleep that matters. The quality of your sleep is a crucial factor that regulates healing and recovery as well as other important processes you'll learn about later.

SLEEP AND CHRONIC STRESS

By now you are probably tired of hearing about the stress response and the autonomic nervous system. Well, it's a factor in sleep too. We're not going to go over what the chronic stress cycle is; by now you already know. We will say that the chronic stress cycle is a major reason why so many Americans have trouble sleeping.

Regardless of what causes the stress response, poor sleep is usually among the consequences. Even worse, poor sleep is a two-way street. We all know that stressors can make sleeping difficult. You may feel tired and constantly fatigued, but stress hormones may keep you constantly on edge. What you may not know is that poor sleep can, in turn, be a stressor itself, which adds to Neuro-Imbalance *(Leproult et al. 1997, 865–70; Vgontzas et al. 1999, 205–15)*.

In fact both sleep disturbances and lack of sleep have been shown to increase the stimulation of the sympathetic nervous system (the *effort and activity* part of the autonomic system) resulting in more stress and less healing *(McEwen 2006, S20–3)*.

And that's not good for anyone.

IMPORTANCE OF DEEP SLEEP—IT'S ABOUT THE QUALITY NOT THE QUANTITY.

It should be pretty clear by now that sleep quality is just as important as sleep duration. Now it's time to define what we mean by *quality sleep*. Quality sleep occurs when the body is able to progress through the natural stages of sleep and spend adequate time in deep sleep (also known as *slow-wave sleep*). Some very important restorative processes happen throughout the body during phases of deep sleep, including that big pulse in growth hormone secretion you learned about earlier. We'll dig into the specifics of those processes shortly, but first you need a basic understanding of the stages of sleep.

Sleep occurs in four stages. Scientists classify these stages from lightest sleep to deepest sleep: REM sleep (rapid eye movement), non-REM 1 (N1), non-REM 2 (N2), and non-REM 3 (N3). Rapid eye movement (REM) sleep is the lightest stage, and non-REM 3 is the deepest form of sleep (also known as deep sleep or slow-wave sleep).

During the night a healthy person progresses through these stages in cycles, with anywhere from three to five sleep cycles occurring each night. The cycles begin with the lightest REM sleep, and then progress into N1, N2, and N3—spending varying amounts of time in each state. The body can then cycle back upward into lighter sleep by slowly progressing in the other direction (N3, N2, N1, REM), or certain steps may be skipped. The exact pattern varies from person to person and night to night. The important thing is that you spend at least some time in each phase of sleep.

During each phase different restorative processes are happening in the brain and throughout the body. While all stages of sleep are important, the focus of this chapter is on deep sleep (N3), because it's crucial for healing and autonomic balance. It is also the phase that many people do not get enough of.

Many people suffering from autonomic imbalance may not be entering into deep sleep throughout the night. And if they are, they may not be experiencing deep sleep often enough or for long enough. The easiest way to judge if you are getting adequate deep sleep is tracking how you feel in the morning. You can sleep for a full eight or nine hours at night, but with inadequate deep sleep, you may still wake up feeling tired instead of refreshed. There are other factors involved in how you feel when you wake up,* but the amount of deep sleep you get is among the most important.

Why is deep sleep so important for health? Deep sleep is the stage of sleep when the brain is least active. It is in stark

---

* The cycle of sleep you awaken from is an important factor in how you feel in the morning. You may feel groggy if you wake up to an alarm while you are in one of the deeper phases of sleep. It's best to awaken naturally at the end of a sleep cycle using your body's natural morning-time spike in cortisol to wake you up.

contrast to other stages of sleep where the brain is quite active. During deep sleep the body focuses its attention and energy on healing and repairing tissues throughout the body. (Remember the restorative pulse in growth hormone that occurs during this phase?) There is also a shift to parasympathetic stimulation, the *healing and recovery* part of the autonomic nervous system, during this stage.

Parasympathetic stimulation further enhances the body's ability to heal itself. This shift into healing-and-recovery mode is especially important for those with a chronic low back condition. That's why deep sleep is part of our autonomic imbalance reducing protocol. During other phases of sleep, sympathetic stimulation is stronger. So without deep sleep, the strong and restorative nighttime dip into parasympathetic stimulation pictured below is blunted, adding to Neuro-Imbalance and all its nasty side effects.

Balanced Autonomic System

(Neuro-Balance)

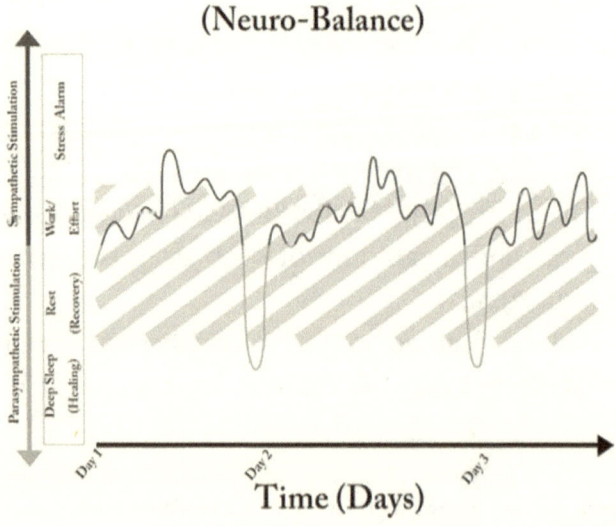

As the graph above illustrates, the parasympathetic stimulation associated with deep sleep is one of the most important tools for balancing the autonomic nervous system. This in turn allows the body to more easily repair damaged cells and subsequent tissues in the body.

Now that you understand why adequate sleep—and especially deep sleep—is so important, it's time to learn how to improve the quality and duration of your sleep. Before we dig into these strategies for better sleep, we want to emphasize the importance of not using medication as a substitute for deep sleep. Medication does not allow you to adequately move through all the stages of sleep. Therefore, you don't spend enough (if any fact you spend any) time in deep, healing sleep.

STRATEGIES FOR GREAT SLEEP

You don't have to sit back and wait for better sleep to happen. There are a number of things you can do to directly improve both sleep duration and quality. Don't ignore these strategies hoping that when your pain goes away you will suddenly start sleeping like a baby. Good sleep is a habit you can get into or out of.

Most back pain patients have suffered from years of poor sleep and have, therefore, developed poor sleeping habits. Oftentimes, they need to relearn how to get great sleep. At the very least, use the following strategies to break your bad sleep cycle. We have found the following to be most effective for improving sleep. You won't be able to implement all these strategies at once, so choose one strategy from near the top of the list, and make your way down.

Unwind Before Bed

Most people lead hectic lives, which will add to any baseline level of stress that they may already be under. High stress is tolerable during the day, but in order to get restful sleep, you need to be relaxed at night.

Relaxing takes time. Most people can't work or do mentally demanding tasks right up until they go to sleep. It takes time to set our worries aside and get relaxed. You need separation between your daily activities and sleep. You should plan on having at least thirty minutes to unwind before bed, but an hour is better. Your relaxation time should not occur in the bedroom. The bedroom, and especially the bed, should be reserved for sleep and intimacy only, no exceptions.

Activities that should be avoided right before bedtime include the following.

- Mentally demanding work
- Discussing emotionally charged issues
- Strenuous physical activity (walking or stretching are exceptions)
- Watching certain TV shows or movies (such as action flicks, thrillers, or mysteries)
- Listening to loud music
- Working on the computer
- Browsing on your cell phone

Here are some things that will better prepare you for bed and allow your body and mind to relax.

- Dim the lights. (Use a dimmer, install lower wattage bulbs in bedroom lamps, or simply use fewer lights.)
- Listen to soothing music.
- Read a calming book (no thrillers or page turners).

- Participate in a hobby or other activity that you find relaxing.
- Write down all of your current thoughts or anxieties—and then let them go.
- Go for a short, relaxing walk.
- Stretch.
- Do some of the breathing exercises that you will learn in the next two sections. (Don't use the respiratory trainer before bed because it is strenuous.)
- Meditate.
- Read something spiritual or uplifting.

SLEEP HYGIENE

Sleep hygiene is a term used to describe how your bedroom and bed is arranged for sleep. Your sleep hygiene can be good or bad, and it has nothing to do with cleanliness. The most important factors in sleep hygiene are light, sound, temperature, mental hygiene, and comfort.

Light—Our bodies are much more sensitive to light than most people realize, and the eyes are not the only part of the body that senses light. Many other cells in the body are sensitive to light, so covering your eyes with an eye mask or sheets won't solve all your problems.

Even the small amount of light coming from charging cell phones, alarm clocks, and other electronics can hamper your ability to sleep. Sensitivities to light vary from person to person, but nearly everyone will benefit from a darker room at night. You may want to consider getting blackout curtains if streetlights or other sources of light come into your bedroom.

Sound—This one is pretty obvious. We all know what it's like to be kept awake by an annoying sound no matter how quiet it may be. If you can control the noise, eliminate it. If a spouse or child is watching TV, listening to music, or playing video games, ask for a noise curfew; it's for your health.

If the noise is out of your control, consider getting a white-noise machine. (These machines play soothing sounds like beach noises or nature sounds.) Another option is to use ear-plugs or get a fan. Earplugs are the most inexpensive solution, but long-term use can cause irritation to the ear.

Temperature—Being too hot or too cold can make it difficult to sleep. Most people prefer a cooler room for sleeping (around seventy degrees). Changing the weight of your bedding to match the season can be a big help. Running the air conditioner in the summer may cost more money, but lost sleep is bad for your health and your productivity, so it may be worth the extra money.

Mental Sleep Hygiene—A racing mind is one of the most common reasons why people have difficulty falling asleep. Giving yourself time to relax and unwind before bed may be enough to help you quiet a racing mind, but for many it's not enough.

One quick-and-easy strategy to quiet your mind is to write down all the things you are worrying about. Many times we mentally run through all the things we want to get done tomorrow while we are lying in bed. Writing your thoughts down on a bedside note pad is a great way to let go of those things. You can easily revisit them in the morning.

Once you have written down all the worries and errands you must take care of the following day, take a few minutes to write down a few things you are grateful for. There is new research showing that having positive thoughts as you fall asleep improves sleep quality and duration and reduces the time it takes to fall asleep in the first place *(Wood et al. 2009, 43–48)*.

Focusing on things for which you are grateful is a powerful tool for getting better sleep. One of the leading researchers in this field, University of California–Davis, psychology professor, Robert Emmons, said it best: "If you want to sleep more soundly, count blessings, not sheep." The simple strategy of keeping a gratitude journal before bed can do wonders for your sleep. Just remember to stick with it. You may not notice the benefits for the first week. This is a long-term sleep improvement strategy; changing your thought patterns before bed will not happen overnight.

Comfort—Comfort is subjective, and no mattress or sleep position will work for everyone. But there are some general guidelines that apply to most people. First off, a worn or sagging mattress must be replaced. It not only ruins your sleep, but it can also cause long-term damage to the back, neck, hips, and shoulders.

Keeping the spine aligned, regardless of your sleeping position, should always be a goal. Side sleepers should use a pillow thick enough to keep the head and neck in line with the spine, preventing the head from tilting down. If necessary an extra pillow between the legs can keep the hips aligned.

If you sleep on your back, you will want a thin pillow under your head to prevent neck problems and a pillow under the knees or calves to take pressure off your low back. (Pillows under the elbows will also make you more comfortable.)

Stomach sleepers should use a very thin pillow to prevent hyperextension of the neck. Stomach sleeping has the most potential to cause problems. If you are a stomach sleeper, you may want to try to break this habit.

Avoid Alcohol, Fluids, and Sugary Snacks before Bed

Alcohol, other beverages, and high-carbohydrate snacks can all cause you to wake up during the night. Alcohol may help you get to sleep faster, but the sleep you get is low quality. Drinking alcohol before bed often causes people to wake up to use the bathroom more frequently and to have lighter, more restless sleep.

Avoid drinking large amounts of anything for about two hours before you go to bed. This will limit the number of times you wake to use the restroom during the night.

Sugary snacks (those high in carbohydrates) raise your blood glucose and eventually cause your blood glucose to drop too low. Low blood glucose during the night causes a cortisol spike that can wake you up, disrupting your sleep cycle.*

Instead, if you want an evening snack, eat a one that's high in protein or fat. A handful of nuts or some celery sticks with almond or cashew butter makes a great bedtime snack. These snacks stick with you throughout the night, causing your body to release a steady amount of glucose into the blood.**

Set a Consistent Schedule

If you are a parent, you know that a child who misses his bedtime will be cranky. Well, we hate to break it to you, but children aren't the only ones who do better with a predictable routine.

---

* Nocturnal cortisol spikes caused by low blood glucose often occur around two or three in the morning.

** High protein snacks before bed will also prevent a spike in cortisol in the early hours of the morning, which will cause many people to wake up. A natural spike in the stress hormone, cortisol, is what wakes us up in the morning.

Setting and following a regular bedtime is extremely important. It may seem strange to set a time that you need to be in bed, but it helps your body form a more consistent daily rhythm. It is equally important to try to wake up at the same time each day.

Set times that will allow you to sleep around eight hours each night. Stick with these times even on weekends and holidays. Getting into a regular sleep pattern will eventually help you feel so much more rested that you'll rarely feel the need to sleep in.

GET THIRTY MINUTES OF MODERATE EXERCISE EACH DAY

Regular exercise can do wonders for your sleep pattern. Light exercise like walking or yard work will help you feel tired at night. It is best if you can exercise in the morning. Remember, you don't have to exercise like an athlete to get sleep benefits. Thirty minutes of light exercise a day is all you need.

The only time you should avoid exercise is right before bed. Exercise tends to stimulate your body and keep it awake. A mild, relaxing walk and stretching are exceptions to the rule for some people, but any other exercise performed before bed can actually keep you awake.

TRY TO GET SOME SUN EACH DAY

Exposure to light helps keep our circadian rhythms in tune with the day-night cycle. Getting exposure to sunlight helps us feel awake during the day and sets our body's internal clock so we know it's bedtime after the sun goes down.

You already learned that it's best to avoid bright lights before bed, but it is important to get exposure to bright light during the day. It's easiest to combine getting sun with getting exercise. If you go for a thirty-minute walk while it's light out, you will be killing two birds with one stone.

Avoid Large Meals Right before Bed

A large meal requires a lot of energy to digest, and for this reason it is best to eat a few hours before bed (unless it's a small protein-based snack).

Get Smart about Naps

Naps are a great way to boost your energy during the day or to make up for lost sleep, but they can be a problem too. If you have trouble falling asleep at night but nap on a regular basis, you need to cut the naps out of your routine. This is especially true if you nap any later than three in the afternoon. These naps may actually be doing more harm than good.

You should also limit a nap should to thirty to forty-five minutes. Any longer and it will almost certainly disrupt your normal sleeping pattern. Fifteen- to twenty-minute naps are ideal. They give you a little boost, but they rarely disrupt your sleep pattern.

Naps are the best way to make up for lost sleep the night before. Going to bed early or sleeping in can throw off your whole schedule. Taking a nap allows you to get a little extra shut-eye while maintaining your normal sleep-wake times.

DO WHAT WORKS

The best sleep strategy is the one that works. All the guidelines above are flexible. If watching a little TV really puts you out and delivers deep, restful sleep, then by all means watch TV. If road noise or chatter from other family members helps you get to sleep, then getting ear plugs won't be useful. Don't be afraid to do what works even if it goes against what works for most people.

This principle is especially true when it comes to sleeping positions. As chiropractors, we see patients all the time with shoulder or neck problems that are partially caused by stomach sleeping or another less-than-perfect sleeping position. But if you are faced with the choice between sleeping an adequate amount of time each night and sleeping in a healthier position, we would recommend getting adequate sleep. *There is no health without restful sleep.*

CHAPTER 18

INLINE POSTURE

There might not seem to be a strong connection between body posture and other chronic conditions, but if you've read this far, then you have learned that the body's systems are incredibly intertwined. Posture is no exception.

Body posture can affect your breathing, digestion, mood, hormones, and—most importantly—the health of your nervous system. (Remember your back pain is a neurological problem.) What's the link between all these factors? You guessed it, the chronic stress response. The chronic stress response affects posture, and conversely posture affects the chronic stress response. For that reason focusing on improving your posture is a great way to reduce Neuro-Imbalance, which is why it's included in the DICE protocol.

Good posture stimulates the parasympathetic (*recovery and healing*) part of the nervous system, which reduces the release of stress hormones and promotes the release of growth and repair hormones including testosterone.* Good posture also affects the other parasympathetic responses like digestion, reduced blood

---

* Testosterone isn't just important for men. In the right amount, testosterone is critical for the health of women as well.

pressure, improved mood, and others. In addition to these positive side effects, good posture has an especially strong
effect on breathing. Bad posture not only sends signals to the brain that promote short shallow breaths, the hunched over position of bad posture physically limits your ability to take deep, full breaths. Good posture allows you to use your diaphragm to breathe more deeply and get more oxygen into your body.

When you combine adequate oxygen, good digestion, and parasympathetic stimulation, you have a recipe for neurological healing. This is exactly what you need for your low back condition.

On top of all the benefits described above, good posture can make you look five years younger. This is not exactly a health benefit, but we all care how we look, and our self-confidence does affect our mood (which is a health benefit).

This chapter on posture is arranged in four sections. First, we will briefly describe the most common type of bad posture. Then we'll cover the ways proper posture benefits your health. Next we will describe exactly what proper posture is. (It's a bit different for everyone.) And lastly we will teach you a few simple exercises you can do at home that will put you on a fast track to good posture and quicker healing.

1. Head-Forward Posture

Although there are many different types of bad posture, the most common is head-forward posture. Don't let the name mislead you. Head-forward posture affects the whole spine not just the head. (The forward head position is just the most noticeable aspect.)

Head-forward posture affects the whole body, including the feet, but for simplicity we will limit this discussion to the areas above the pelvis. In many cases when you align the spine properly, the legs, knees, and feet tend to correct themselves, especially if you are being checked for neuromechanical balance.

People who suffer from head-forward posture rotate their pelvis forward. This causes the lumbar spine (the lowest part of the spine) to have too much forward curve (making your belly stick out). The exaggerated lumbar curve forces your body to curve the thoracic spine (the middle part) backward in order to stay balanced.

To compensate for everything that's going on below, the cervical spine (the neck) and head are thrust forward. This situation is like a stack of blocks arranged in a zigzag pattern. It will stand, but it isn't the most stable arrangement.

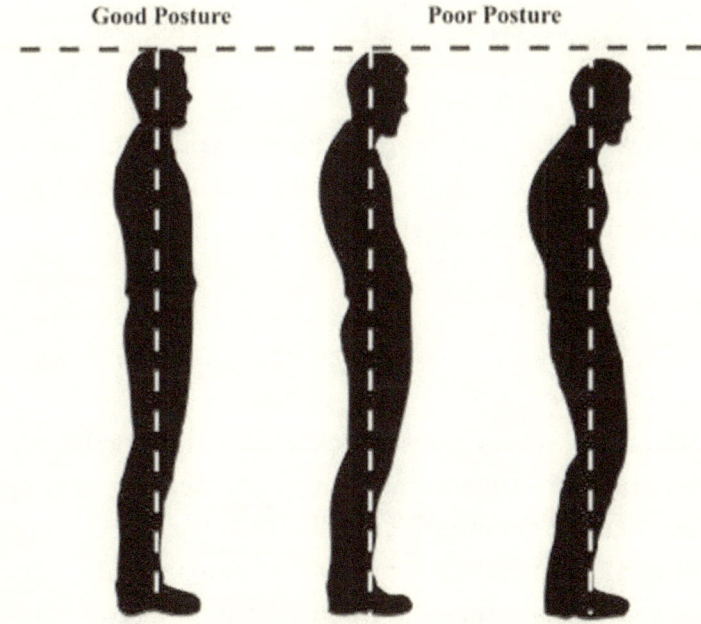

Good Posture   **Poor Posture**

Proper posture is like a stack of blocks that is almost perfectly aligned up and down. It is by no means a straight line. (We are designed for movement not for standing perfectly straight.) But it is much more stable than head-forward posture.

Remember, just like a stack of blocks, posture is nothing more than a balancing act. Head-forward posture is your body's best attempt to stay upright. Unfortunately, this promotes disc degeneration, arthritis, and the chronic stress response.

Luckily there is a better, healthier way to balance your body. And after some practice it will actually require the use of less energy, give you more energy, and make you feel and look better.

Believe it or not, most of us are born with great posture. But after twelve or more years of hunching over a desk in school, many more years of work (using your back or bent over an office desk), hundreds of hours driving cars, and in general sitting for most of our lives, our naturally good posture slowly erodes, and a new hunched-over posture becomes our norm. Stressors only add to our tendency to develop bad posture.

Don't worry though; you can regain your long-lost good posture through practice. Your brain still knows how to properly align your spine; you just have to remind it how.

WHY WORRY ABOUT HEAD-FORWARD POSTURE

Head-forward posture causes muscle fatigue, tension headaches, tingling hands and fingers, back pain, shoulder pain, neck pain, and other health problems. It contributes to various chronic diseases by stimulating the sympathetic nervous system, preventing proper deep breathing, and perpetuating Neuromechanical Imbalance and in turn the chronic stress cycle.

2. How Good Posture Heals

Posture and Breathing

In order to take slow, deep breaths, you must have good posture and be neuromechanically balanced. A recent study showed that people with head-forward posture had weaker respiratory muscles than those with proper alignment *(Kapreli 2009.)* Breathing and posture go hand in hand. Weak posture equals weak breathing, and strong posture equals strong breathing.

If you suffer from head-forward posture, then you will likely have a hard time breathing from your diaphragm. The extra curvature of your thoracic spine causes your rib cage to drop lower and to put more pressure on your stomach.

This position limits the amount your diaphragm is able to move. If your diaphragm can't access its full range of motion, you will naturally compensate by taking rapid, shallow breaths using only your upper lungs instead of your more efficient lower lungs.

As you will learn in the chapter on complete breathing (the *C* in the DICE protocol), taking quick, shallow breaths with only your upper lungs stimulates your sympathetic nervous system and increases your chronic stress response, which in turn slows down healing. Remember, good posture—and the deep, full breaths that come with it—stimulate the healing side of your nervous system (the parasympathetic nervous system). A 2010 study showed that even brief, two-minute changes in posture can lower cortisol and boost testosterone secretion *(Carney et al. 2010, 1363–8).* This study demonstrates the powerful effect posture can have on the hormonal component of the stress response. Additionally, for many of us, better posture is the easiest route to deeper diaphragmatic breathing.

GOOD POSTURE FOR A HEALTHY BRAIN

Believe it or not, having good posture is good for your brain. Do you recall the charge for your brain? Mechanoreceptors are responsible for providing the proper stimulation for your nerves to stay alive and healthy. Your brain simply requires constant stimulation.

Where does posture fit in? The muscles that cause good posture are stimulated by a part of your brain called the pontomedulary reticular formation (PMRF for short). Since neurological stimulation is a two-way street, having good posture also stimulates the PMRF. (Signals don't just go out from the brain, they go back into the brain as well, remember?)

Bad posture sends signals to your brain too, but it sends the wrong kind of signals. Having an underactive (or weak) PMRF can result in poor posture, and poor posture can also weaken your PMRF. This is true even if your bad posture was caused by life habits instead of a neurological condition.

At the end of the day, it doesn't really matter if your bad posture is from a weak (under-firing) PMRF or if you simply have bad posture due to years of work. Both problems can be treated with specific posture exercises that "wake up" the PMRF and get it working better. Once your PMRF is stronger, it will start activating the muscles that lead to good posture (deep multifidi) without you having to think about it. This doesn't happen overnight, but it does work.

So what have we learned so far? Good posture improves balance and promotes proper breathing. And, perhaps most importantly, practicing good posture is a safe and easy way to fire up the PMRF.

Why is firing up the PMRF so important? One of the many functions of the PMRF is to act as a kind of governor for the sympathetic nervous system. A weak PMRF allows the sympathetic nervous system to go unchecked, which allows the stress response to dominate your body adding to autonomic imbalance.

Practicing good posture and regularly doing targeted posture exercises will help you throttle down the stress response.

POSTURE AND DIGESTION

Posture affects digestion in two very important ways. First, good posture stimulates the parasympathetic nervous system—which, as you know, is often referred to as the rest-and-digest part of the autonomic nervous system. It gets this name because the parasympathetic nervous system promotes digestion by stimulating the release of various digestive enzymes and stomach acid and stimulates the directional movement of food through the intestines. In contrast the sympathetic nervous system does the exact opposite *(Thompson and Richelson and Malagelada 1982, 1200–6)*.

The second negative effect bad posture has on digestion is a bit less complex. When you carry yourself with bad posture, your intestines pile up on the pelvic floor restricting proper flow of digesting food *(Cailliet 1987, 53)*. In contrast, with good posture, the intestines are held in proper placement so that food can move through the GI tract easily.

POSTURE, MOOD, AND CONFIDENCE

It has long been known that posture affects the way people perceive and judge you. People with better posture are judged as more attractive and confident, while those with bad posture are more likely to be seen as less attractive and less confident.

Newer research is showing that good posture not only affects the way others perceive you, but it also directly affects the way you feel about yourself (regardless of what others think). The same posture study we talked about earlier showed that strong posture increased a person's sense of power *(Carney et al. 2010, 1363–8)*. Better posture can boost your confidence in yourself physically (feeling better about the way you look) and mentally (feeling more confident in your own thoughts and decisions). Good posture also lowers the amount of the stress hormone, cortisol, produced by your body.

With all that you know about good posture, how can you not believe it's always worthy of improvement?

3. What Is Good Posture?

Our bodies were designed to move efficiently. Posture is the body's attempt to keep us upright in the strongest, most stable and efficient way possible. Because every person is unique, good posture varies from person to person. Despite these differences there are some characteristics that everyone with good posture will share.

We are all designed to have our ankles, knees, hips, shoulders, and ears roughly lined up vertically.

This probably comes as no surprise to you. We all instinctively know what good posture looks like. (It's one of the major ways we subconsciously interpret attractiveness.) The problem is that few of us have a realistic view of our own posture.

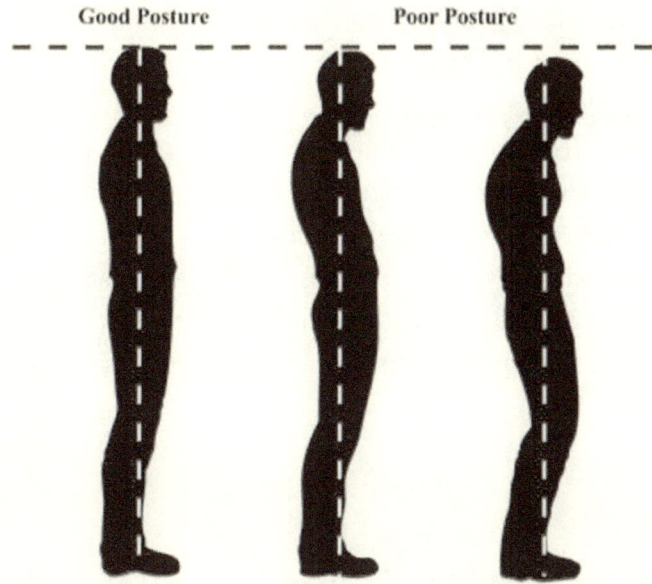

Good Posture   Poor Posture

Aside from looking in the bathroom mirror in the mornings, we rarely get a good look at ourselves, especially when we are doing normal daily activities.

It is all too common for people to think they have better posture than they actually do. For this reason one of the exercises in this section asks you to have someone take a front and side posture picture of you. This will help you align what you think your posture looks like, with what it actually looks like.

EXERCISES FOR GOOD POSTURE

Do you recall when your mother or grandmother always told you to sit up straight or to stop slouching? These instructions probably didn't fix your poor posture. You straightened up for a minute or two but quickly fell back into a slouched position.

Most people can force themselves into good posture when they think about it, but the reality is we cannot spend the whole day thinking about our posture.

The real trick is retraining your brain so that you eventually sit and stand with better posture without even thinking about it.

There are two types of exercises that will help you do this. Some are designed to make you more aware of your posture, so you notice your bad posture more often. The others are designed to stimulate the part of your brain that keeps you upright.

PELVIC ROTATION

The goal of this exercise is to make you aware of any excessive curvature of your lower back. Along with giving you awareness, it will teach you to use the muscles that remove that excessive curvature. When the lower back (lumbar spine) has the proper amount of curvature, your mid and upper back will be able to return to their natural curvature much more easily *(Weiniger 2008, 5–8)*.

PELVIC ROTATIONS WITH WALL

1. Stand with your back against a wall. Your heels should be a foot away from the wall and your knees should be straight but not fully locked out.
2. Your buttocks, shoulders, and the back of your head should all be pressed against the wall. If you can't get your shoulder and head against the wall at the same time don't worry, this exercise should help with your head-forward posture. In the meantime keep your shoulders

against the wall and look straight ahead with your head
level.

3. Relax your arms so that your hands are at your sides.
Move your hands a few inches away from your body, and
press the back of your hands into the wall.

4. While keeping your knees extended (straight), breathe in
and arch your back as slowly as you can. Keep your buttock, shoulders, and head against the wall.

5. When your back is arched as much as possible, start
breathing out while slowly pressing the small of your
back against the wall. Get your low back as close to the
wall as possible by trying to pull your belly button in
toward the wall. You will have to flex your abdominals
to do this properly. (Note that your buttocks may move
away from the wall, which is fine).

6. Repeat this forward and backward rotation of the pelvis
five times. It is important that you do this as slowly as
possible and focus on how it feels. Doing this exercise
slowly teaches you how to consciously control some of
the posture muscles you subconsciously use all the time.

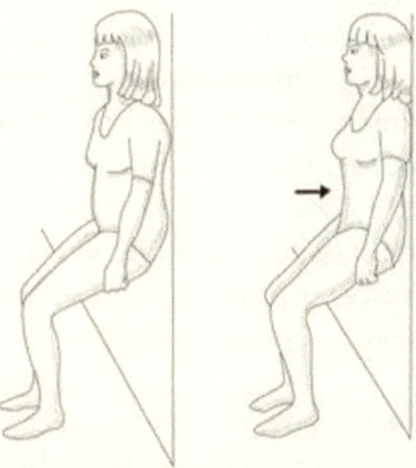

This exercise should be done daily. Good posture is built from the ground up. The only way to eliminate head-forward posture, and the discomfort and pain it causes, is to remove the excess curvature of the lower back. Only when the excess curvature of the lower back is reduced can the other exercises presented below start bringing your head back into alignment.

Unlock Your Knees

Oftentimes we stand with our knees locked. Locking your knees for long periods of time—for example, when standing over the sink doing dishes—is a recipe for bad posture. When the knees lock, the pelvis rotates forward, starting the chain reaction that results in bad posture *(Novak 2006, 59)*. In addition bending over with your knees locked forces you to bend at the waist not at the hips. This type of bending promotes bad posture and back injuries.

Learning to unlock your knees while standing is not strenuous or difficult, you just have to break a very ingrained habit. There are no exercises for this. It's all about awareness. Simply unlock your knees whenever you think about your posture.

There is a lot of confusion about what locking your knees looks like. For most people, when the knee joint is fully extended, the knee actually bends slightly behind you. This is what we call being *locked*. When your leg is straight, you can usually extend the knee just a little bit more. It's this little extra extension that causes the problem. Just realize that not locking your knees does not mean that you have to stand around with your knees bent.

If you have trouble remembering to unlock your knees, write a reminder on a note, and put it above the bathroom sink and above the kitchen sink. These are two places where everyone tends to stand in one place for several minutes a day.

HEAD BACK

This is one of the simplest exercises for good posture.

1. Clasp your hands behind your head (interlocking your fingers).
2. While looking straight ahead, cup the back of your head with your clasped hands.
3. Keep your elbows wide and back.
4. Try to push your head back while resisting that movement with your clasped hands.
5. Hold the pressure for five seconds and then release for five seconds. Repeat three times.

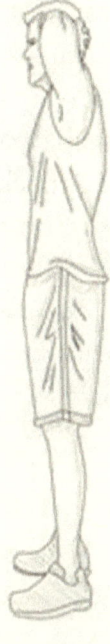

When doing this exercise, move your head back with slow steady pressure—no jerking or straining. And exert only as much pressure against your hands as is comfortable *(Novak 2006, 24)*.

GOOD-MORNING STRETCH

Despite its name, this quick stretch can be done any time of day. Here's how.

1. Stand tall with your best posture, and look straight ahead with your arms at your side.
2. Begin to look upward as you take a deep breath.
3. As you begin to breathe in, lift your arms in a circular motion from your sides until they meet above your head (like you are making a snow angel).
4. Time your breathing so that you have taken in as much air as you can when your hands meet above your head. When your lungs are full, you should be looking up as much as is comfortable, and your hands should be together or slightly crossing one another.
5. Now slowly exhale while you lower your arms to your side and your head goes back to level.
6. Repeat this exercise five times.

This is one of our favorite exercises because it includes both a posture exercise and a breathing exercise *(Adams 2011)*. That means fewer exercises to worry about throughout the day. Make this part of your daily routine.

WALL W'S

This is a simple but powerful exercise that fires up the PMRF and gets your brain to start sending good posture signals to your back and neck muscles.

1. Stand with your back flat against a wall. (Your knees should be bent to achieve this.)
2. Hold your arms up like a football referee signaling a touchdown, then bend your elbows to the level of your shoulders.
3. Rotate your palms forward and fingers backward.
4. Now press your elbows and fingers against the wall behind you squeezing your shoulder blades together.
5. Hold this position for three seconds.
6. Bring your hands in front of you, maintaining the elbow position.
7. Repeat the process ten times.

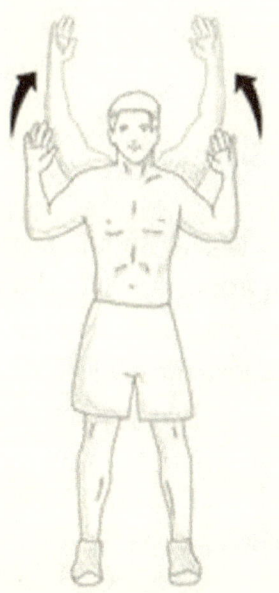
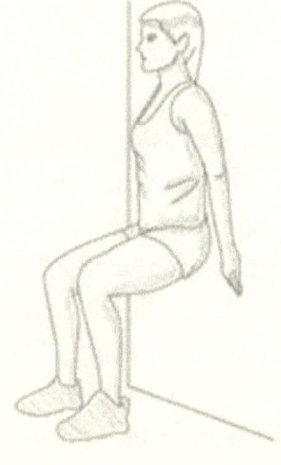

With this exercise you want to focus on squeezing your shoulder blades together. Also be sure to keep your head level, the back of your head against the wall, and your pelvis tucked under so that your low back is as flat against the wall as possible. If you have severe head-forward posture and cannot get or keep the back of your head against the wall, hold your head back as far as you can without pain. (Don't look up and tilt your head back to get it close to the wall; it's important that your head remains level, eyes looking forward.)

EXERCISES WITH A RESISTANCE BAND

If you have an exercise band, there are some great posture exercises you can start doing right away that are easy and effective. If you don't have an exercise band, you don't need to rush out and get one. Stick to the exercises above for a few weeks. Once you have mastered all the exercises above, buy a band and incorporate the techniques below into your routine.

SHOULDER-BLADE SQUEEZE

The rhomboids are muscles that attach your shoulder blade to your spine. In a healthy person with good posture, the rhomboids keep the shoulders opened up and prevent them from rolling toward the front. If you have lost the muscle tone that keeps your shoulders back, this exercise will help you strengthen those muscles *(Novak 2006, 32)*.

1. Start by grasping the band with each hand. There should be eight inches of band between each hand.

2. Hold your hands in front of you. Keep your elbows bent at a ninety-degree angle.
3. While keeping your elbows up and your hands level with your armpits, pull your elbows backward like you are squeezing something between your shoulder blades.
4. With your shoulder blades squeezed together and your elbows still at ninety degrees, hold the tension for two seconds, then relax and rest for two seconds.
5. Repeat five times.

As you progress in strength, move your hold on the band closer together to decrease the space between each hand and increase the tension.

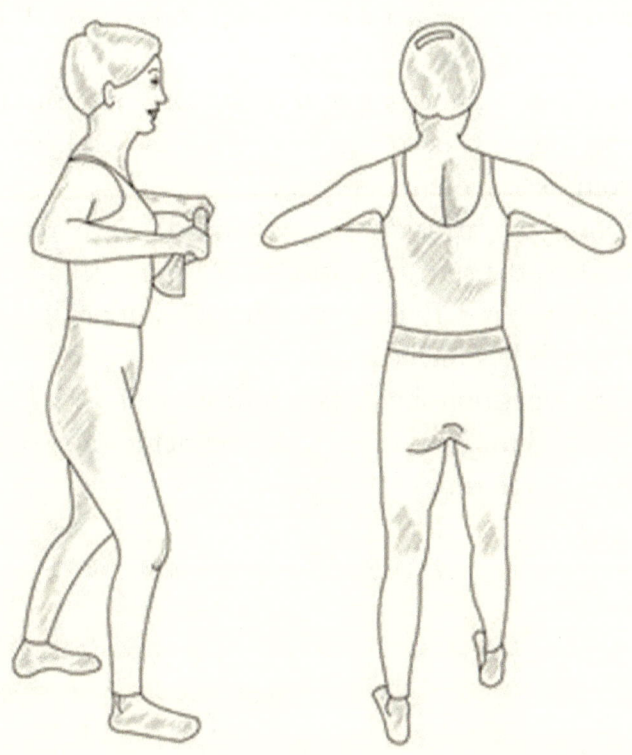

HEAD RETRACTIONS WITH BAND

This exercise really fires up the PMRF. The name of this exercise is a bit misleading. You aren't actually going to be moving your head at all. You are simply going to be resisting the forward pressure of the exercise band. This requires that you use the muscles that hold your head back.

1. Start by grasping the exercise band with about eighteen inches of band between your hands.
2. Move the band that is between your hands behind your head (not your neck).
3. With your elbows in front of you, look straight ahead, move your head back attempting to create a double chin, and stretch the band by moving your hands straight out in front of you.
4. While slowly moving your hands forward, resist the pressure on your head with your neck muscles. Try to keep your head from moving at all.
5. Once your arms are fully extended, slowly retract them back to the starting position. Try not to let any slack get into the band. Even at the starting position, it should still be slightly stretched.
6. One repetition should take four seconds. Bring your head forward for two seconds, and retract it for two seconds.
7. Repeat ten times.

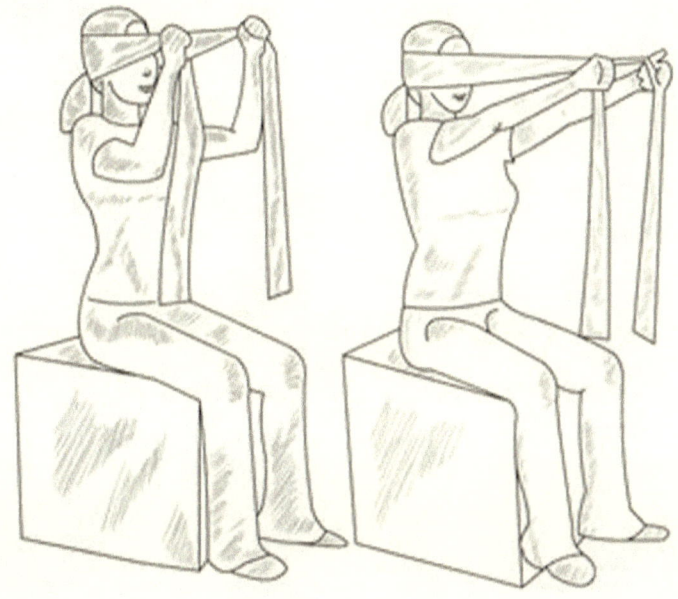

You can adjust the tension on the band (making this exercise more or less difficult) by increasing or decreasing the space between your hands.

CHAPTER 19

COMPLETE BREATHING

Few things are more crucial to overall health than proper breathing. Proper breathing is an especially powerful tool for lowering chronic stress response and unlocking your body's natural healing power (by increasing parasympathetic activity). But unless you suffer from a breathing-related condition, you likely give little thought to the way you breathe and how it affects your health.

That's about to change. This chapter describes exactly why proper breathing is so important to your health and your energy levels and, more specifically, how it can lower the chronic stress response and aid overall body recovery. You will also learn how to retrain your breathing habits to maximize all the health-boosting side benefits of proper breathing.

BREATHING AND HEALTH

Let's start with the basics. Breathing supplies all the cells in your body with oxygen, which is crucial for every function in the body. When air enters the lungs, oxygen is absorbed into the small capillary blood vessels of the lungs. From there your circulatory system (blood vessels and arteries) carries oxygen throughout the body.

Every cell in your body requires a regular supply of oxygen to survive. Nerve cells are especially sensitive to slight variations in blood oxygen concentration in the blood stream. Increasing your blood oxygenation (amount of oxygen in the blood given as a percentage) is one of the fundamental ways to promote healing within the body. Proper breathing can boost low blood oxygenation.

Proper breathing is the simplest way to increase the amount of oxygen in oxygen-starved areas of the body. The best part is that you won't have to take any drugs or carry around an oxygen tank.

BENEFITS OF PROPER BREATHING

Proper breathing has two very important benefits to you.

First, it allows you to breathe into the lower lobe of each lung. The lower lobes of the lungs have more capillary blood vessels than the upper lobes. If you utilize the lower lobes of your lungs, you will be able to absorb more oxygen from each breath.

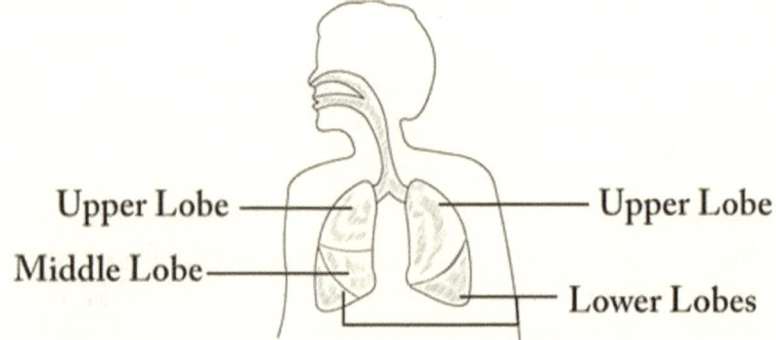

Using the lower lobes of the lungs makes your breathing much more efficient. When you breathe into the lower portions of the lungs, you are essentially getting more bang for your buck with each breath.

Second, proper breathing promotes a balanced nervous system by stimulating your parasympathetic (*recovery and healing*) nervous system, which reduces Neuro-Imbalance. As you may remember, the parasympathetic nervous system is in charge of healing. It's the part of the nervous system that opposes the sympathetic (*fight or flight*) nervous system. In order to promote healing throughout the body, you need to stimulate your parasympathetic nervous system as much as possible. Proper breathing is an easy and effective way to do just that.

The importance of breathing in establishing and maintaining a balanced nervous system cannot be understated. In fact Andrew Weil, MD, a world renowned, Harvard trained, leader in integrative medicine, has this to say on the subject of breathing,

...many common health problems, including irregular heart rhythms, high blood pressure, poor circulation, stomach and intestinal disorders, and more, have as their underlying cause an imbalance in the involuntary nervous system. Although conventional physicians often prescribe drugs to correct such imbalances, breathing techniques alone can often do the job, serving as a natural tranquilizer for your nervous system, gradually and consistently giving it information that can harmonize body function (Weil 2005, 14).

Poor breathing habits are associated with imbalance in the autonomic nervous system *(Courtney and Cohen and van Dixhoorn 2011, 38–44)*. This is measured through heart-rate variability (HRV). Heart rate is heavily influenced by breathing patterns; this phenomenon is referred to as the *respiratory sinus arrhythmia*. Heart rate and breathing are tied together for several very important reasons that we won't get into here. All you need to know is that this coordination promotes proper circulation and oxygenation of blood throughout the circulatory system.

Breathing is the easiest way to enable healthy heart-rate variability. Managing heart-rate variability is a well-known strategy for self-regulating the stress response and the negative physiological responses that result *(Paul and Garg 2012, 131–44)*. For that reason developing good breathing habits can dampen the chronic stress response and consequently lower Neuro-Imbalance.

You cannot eliminate chronic stress from your life, but you can reduce it and the toll it takes on your body. Using breathing exercises that stimulate the parasympathetic nervous system is the easiest and most effective way to promote healing and reduce the imbalance. In fact you can start the change with just a few breaths. Proper breathing is an included therapy in the DICE protocol because of the quick results it provides along with its power over the chronic stress response.

As we've mentioned earlier, being in a parasympathetic state has a large number of benefits for the body. First and foremost, parasympathetic stimulation dilates (opens up) the capillaries, arteries, and blood vessels of the body. This opening up of the vascular system increases the blood flow throughout your body *(Lee and Campbell 2009, 60)*.

When you combine the opening up of the vascular system with more efficient breathing, the benefit to your body is quite remarkable. More efficient breathing puts more oxygen into your blood. Dilation of the blood vessels and capillaries allows the increased amount of oxygen and other vital nutrients to reach the nerves throughout the body.

Getting highly oxygenated blood into cells is crucial if you want to promote healing. Studies have shown that the availability of oxygen has a direct effect upon every cell's ability to heal.

In addition oxygen is often the limiting factor in the healing process *(Lee and Campbell 2009, 92–4)*. It's no wonder that professional athletes commonly use oxygen therapy to shorten healing times after injuries. Proper breathing has also been proven to lower stress and reduce the risk of heart disease. How's that for side effects?

HOW TO BREATHE PROPERLY

Although it is something we often give little thought to, the body is capable of breathing in a number of different ways. These types of breathing are usually used in different combinations depending on what you are doing. For example we breathe differently for each of the follow activities: talking, sleeping, exercising, eating, working, and resting.

The two main types of breathing are costal breathing and diaphragmatic breathing. Although it is difficult to completely isolate them from each other, one or the other often dominates our breathing pattern.

COSTAL BREATHING

Costal breathing utilizes the expansion of the rib cage to take a breath. There are dozens of muscles that can open up the rib cage and cause your lungs to fill with air. The ribs are able to rotate outward and upward, like lifting the handle on a bucket. Expanding your rib cage fills the lungs with air because the lungs are stuck to the inside of the rib cage. When the rib cage opens up, it stretches the lungs and causes them to fill with air.

Costal Breathing

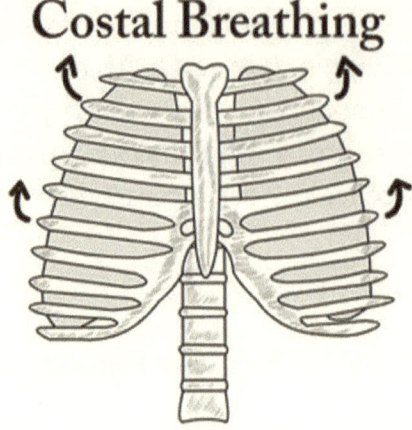

The Ribs Rotate Upward & Outward Stretching
the Lungs to Draw in Air

Costal breathing (breathing with the ribs) primarily fills the upper portion of the lungs with air. As you know, the upper portions of the lungs are less efficient at absorbing oxygen than the lower parts of the lungs. This means that if you breathe primarily using your ribs, you will need to take a breath more often, and you will get less oxygen out of each breath.

DIAPHRAGMATIC BREATHING

Diaphragmatic breathing uses a muscle called the diaphragm to stretch the lungs and draw in air. The diaphragm is shaped like an umbrella and is attached to the spine, the perimeter of the lower ribs, and the sternum. The center of the diaphragm (top of the umbrella) is attached indirectly to the lower portion of the lungs.*

---

* Each lung is attached to an inner pleural membrane and the inner membrane sticks and slides with an outer pleural membrane. The outer pleural membrane is attached to the diaphragm.

In its resting position, the diaphragm is stretched upward by the lungs. When the diaphragm contracts through inspiration, it moves downward (toward your pelvis) stretching the lungs like an accordion and causing you to take a breath. Because the diaphragm is connected with the lower lobes of the lungs, it stretches the lower lobes of the lungs more than the upper lobes. This results in more air moving into the lower lobes of the lungs.

The lower lobes of the lungs have more capillaries to absorb oxygen, so a diaphragmatic breath is more efficient than a costal breath.

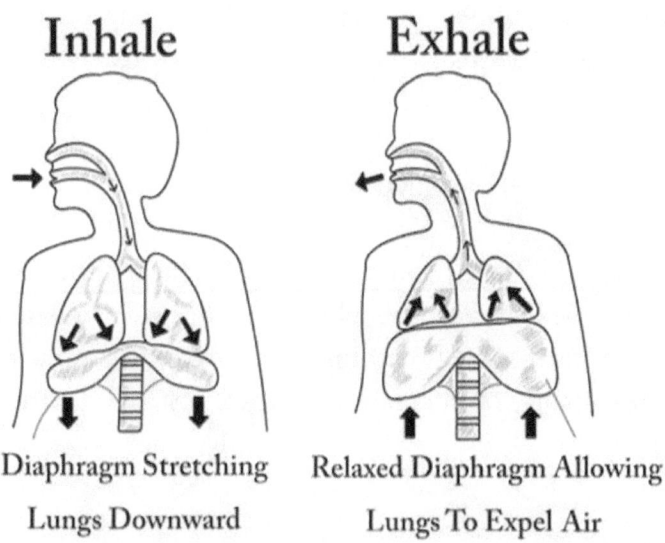

Inhale	Exhale
Diaphragm Stretching Lungs Downward	Relaxed Diaphragm Allowing Lungs To Expel Air

Both types of breathing are important, and an inability to use one or the other will certainly have a negative impact on your health. Breathing primarily with short, shallow breaths will stimulate the sympathetic nervous system and will increase your chronic stress response.

The most common breathing restriction we see in our office is rib immobility. This immobility can come from scar-tissue adhesions due to old injury, tight muscles from years of stress, mechanical imbalances, or simply a lack of exercise.

However, most people who take shallow, frequent breaths don't have any breathing restriction. For now we're going to assume that the primary reason most people take short, shallow breaths is that they are simply in the habit of doing so. This bad habit develops over a person's lifetime as a result of various factors: working hunched over a computer, sitting in uncomfortable office chairs, driving for long hours, slouching on a couch, and experiencing stressful daily events.

In order to take advantage of all the benefits of proper breathing, you will need to turn your shallow, frequent breaths into slow deep breaths.

RELEARNING HOW TO BREATHE

This section will teach you how to break the shallow breathing habit by first learning to feel what type of breath you are taking. You'll then learn some breathing exercises and a simple training program to help you increase the efficiency and depth of your breathing.

LEARN TO NOTICE YOUR BREATH

In order to control your breath, you must become aware of it. This is a pretty straightforward process. Simply take a moment, and notice how you are breathing. Once you become aware of your breath, you almost always start to change it. That's OK; just keep breathing. Try to notice how it feels and where your breath is going.

Here are some things to look for.

1. Are your shoulders moving up and down with each breath?
2. Do you feel your rib cage opening up as you breathe?
3. Place a hand on your lower ribs and take a breath; now place your hand on the upper ribs below your armpit and take a breath. Where did you feel more movement?
4. Does your stomach move in when you inhale, or does it move out?

Please perform the observations described above before you read on.

Based on your answers to these questions, you can get an idea of how you are breathing. You may have to do this a couple of times. We often dramatically change our normal breathing cycle when we think about it too much. Wait a few hours, and do the exercise again to see if your results are the same. We are constantly changing our breathing patterns, but everyone has a baseline they return to when relaxed. Use the points below to self assess your breathing habits.

1. If your shoulders moved up and down when you take a normal resting breath, you are using your ribs to breathe.
2. If you felt a lot of movement in any area of your ribs, you are primarily using your ribs to breathe.
3. If your stomach moved in while you inhaled, you are definitely using your ribs to breathe. If your stomach moved out as you inhaled, you are using your diaphragm at least partially to breathe.
4. If you felt little movement in your ribs, you weren't moving your shoulders up and down, and your stomach moved out when you inhaled, you are mostly using your diaphragm to breathe. (Those are good sign and what we tell all our patients to strive for.)

Before going any further, we want to stress that we are dealing with how you breathe while resting. If you are exercising or being active, it is perfectly normal to use your ribs and your diaphragm to breathe. Breathing with your ribs is not always bad. In fact later on we'll describe an exercise that strengthens both types of breathing and has huge benefits for people suffering from the chronic stress response. Focusing on diaphragmatic breathing while resting is simply a great tool to stimulate the parasympathetic nervous system and increase your breathing efficiency.

Hopefully after performing this breath-awareness exercise, you have a better idea of how you naturally breathe. It might be helpful to write down some notes on what you noticed. The goal of the exercises in this chapter is to modify the way you breathe while resting. To track your progress, it is very helpful to have a benchmark to look back on.

In order to change the way you breathe, you need to become conscious of your breathing as often as possible. It may seem like a lot of work, but it is crucial to promote healing and repair. It will take some time, but the more you think about it, the more you will be able to transform your breathing. The more often you are able to change your breath from rapid and shallow to slow and deep, the more quickly it will become a habit. This in turn will help the healing process and give you more energy!

BREATHING EXERCISES

The breathing exercises that you will be taught are simple and require very little time. They are so easy you can perform them while sitting on your couch.

We recommend you find some quiet time with no distraction the first couple of times you try these exercises. After the initial few sessions, you can start performing these exercises while watching TV, while driving, at work, and pretty much any other time you are not doing something strenuous. OK, enough talk, let's get down to business.

The first exercise is designed to get you to relax and focus on exhaling slowly. Exhaling slowly is the real secret to stimulating your parasympathetic nervous system.

For this exercise you should find a quiet place where you can sit in a comfortable chair without being disturbed for five to ten minutes. Sit with your back reasonably straight. You don't have to be as straight as a board, but you want to avoid slouching, which will limit your ability to breathe freely.

Breathing exercises can sometimes make you feel a bit light-headed. If you experience this—especially the first few times you perform this breathing exercise—don't worry. However, if you do feel light-headed, stop the exercise and return to your normal breathing for a minute or two, then try the exercise again. After a few sessions, you should no longer experience this problem.

This exercise works best if you focus on initiating each breath with your diaphragm. So before we get started, here are a few tips on breathing using your diaphragm.

The best way to ensure that your breathing pattern is dominated by your diaphragm is to focus on pushing your belly button out while you inhale. Place a hand on your stomach so you can get a feel for it. We will be taking fairly deep breaths during this exercise, so you will be using your ribs too, but make sure you start the breath with your diaphragm pushing your stomach out. When you can't breathe any deeper by pushing your stomach out, go ahead and start to raise your shoulders, which will open up your rib cage.

By using this technique, you will get air deep into the most efficient part of your lungs first. Oftentimes, if you inhale with your ribs first, it is difficult to fill the lower lungs using the diaphragm.

This exercise is nothing more than a regulated breathing pattern that is optimized to increase your oxygen intake and stimulate your parasympathetic nervous system.

We will use simple counting to measure our inhale time, the pauses, and the exhale time. For this exercise you are going to inhale deeply for four seconds. You will then hold this air in your lungs for seven seconds. Next you will slowly and steadily exhale for eight seconds *(Weil 2005, 15)*. This will require you to exhale much more slowly than you inhale to avoid running out of breath before the seven seconds are up. To help you relax, you may close your eyes for this exercise.

Breathing Exercise
Inhale...1...2...3...4 Pause...1...2...3...4...5...6...7
Exhale slowly...1...2...3...4...5...6...7...8
Inhale...1...2...3...4 Pause...1...2...3...4...5...6...7
Exhale slowly...1...2...3...4...5...6...7...8
Repeat this for a total of ten breaths.

If this seems nearly impossible for you initially, you can also reduce the counts to three counts for an inhale and six counts for an exhale until this becomes easy for you to perform.

How do you feel? Most people feel very relaxed after this simple exercise. That feeling of relaxation is accompanied by a boost in your immune system, an opening up of your vascular system, and a boost in cellular healing throughout the body. Even if you don't feel any differently, you have just lowered your chronic stress.

This exercise can be done one or more times daily. The more you use this exercise the better. It usually requires a bit more peace and quiet than the next exercise (which can be done anywhere), but you should feel comfortable using it in almost any daily situation. It can also help stop a spike in your sympathetic nervous system, which is brought on by a stressful situation.

This next exercise is called the ten-second breath. Each breathing cycle (a complete breath consists of an inhale and an exhale) doesn't have to take ten seconds, but ten seconds should be your goal. Why ten seconds? Research has shown that reducing your number of breaths from the average of twelve to fifteen per minute to six breaths per minute has huge health benefits.

Taking only six (longer, deeper) breaths per minute can increase your total oxygen intake by around 15 percent and can boost your blood-oxygen saturation by around 7 percent *(Lee and Campbell 2009, 95)*. So even if you achieve half of the benefits seen by the researchers of the ten-second breath, you will still see significant results and bring your blood oxygenation into the optimum healing range of 98–100 percent. Although a few percentage points may not seem like much, your oxygen-sensitive nerve cells (and all other cells) know the difference.

Of course you can't just start taking six breaths per minute all of a sudden. It requires a bit of training. You will build up to this rate over the course of a few weeks. To start with, you can focus on six- or eight-second breaths. Before you know it, you'll be down to six breaths per minute, helping to put your body's blood oxygenation level into the optimum healing zone, and feeling very relaxed and energized.

For this exercise you simply breathe in for the same number of counts as you exhale with a one-count pause when your lungs are full and also when they are empty *(Lee and Campbell 2009, 52–3)*. For example, you may want to start with breathing in for three seconds then exhaling for three seconds.

Inhale 1...2...3 Pause

Exhale 1...2...3 Pause

Inhale 1...2...3 Pause

Exhale 1...2...3 Pause

When this pace is comfortable and you do not experience any light-headedness, simply count to four for each inhale and exhale (eight-second breath). When eight-second breaths are comfortable, you can progress to ten-second breaths.

This exercise can be used anytime during the day. You should aim to practice it whenever you think about it (while waiting in lines, doing laundry, watching TV, driving, etc.). The more often you use it, the more often your blood oxygenation concentration will be in the optimum range.

RESPIRATORY MUSCLE TRAINER

This last exercise uses a unique breathing trainer that has been proven in many studies to strengthen the muscles used for breathing. Strengthening the respiratory muscles used for breathing has many benefits.

As we age our respiratory muscles tend to weaken and get smaller. This can prevent older patients from taking full, deep breaths. Using a respiratory muscle trainer strengthens these muscles and can increase the maximum amount of air you can inhale during a deep breath.

Respiratory training has another major benefit. Strengthening the respiratory muscles has been shown to reduce the incidence of shortness of breath in older individuals. Many of our older patients experience shortness of breath during low intensity exercise such as walking or shopping. We also have had a number of patients who experience shortness of breath on occasion during regular household chores.

Shortness of breath can have a serious impact on your quality of life. Respiratory training will enable you to do more of the things you used to do without worrying about shortness of breath—things like grocery shopping, walking the dog, and playing with the grandkids.

Shortness of breath stimulates the sympathetic nervous system, which reduces blood circulation to the limbs. Every time you are short of breath, you are reducing the blood flow to the nerve cells *(Chiappa et al. 2008, 1663–71)*.

Respiratory training strengthens your respiratory muscles making them more resistant to fatigue. This results in less shortness of breath during moderate exercise. It also means that daily activities and moderate exercise will not result in reduced blood flow to your limbs.

Now that you understand the importance of respiratory training, let's take a look at how to train your respiratory muscles.

We recommend that patients purchase a respiratory trainer called the BreathBooster®. Although most respiratory trainers will work just fine, we have found the BreathBooster® to be easy to use and inexpensive. It is a simple device that creates resistance when you inhale and exhale through it.*

The idea is simple; by making it more difficult to inhale, your respiratory muscles will get stronger. Study after study has proven that the respiratory muscles do in fact get stronger after this kind of exercise (even in older individuals).

---

* For information on where you can buy a BreathBooster® see section four.

The training program is not difficult; simply follow the instructions below.

1. Start with the BreathBooster® at the easiest setting. (The entire aperture should be visible.)
2. Make sure you are sitting with good, upright posture.
3. Place the mouthpiece in your mouth so that the two wings rest between your teeth and gums, and then grip the two bits between your teeth to form an airtight seal.
4. Draw in a fast, forceful breath through the mouthpiece, and continue to draw in as hard and as fast as you can until your lungs are completely full, taking care not to breathe in through your nose. Make sure you straighten your back and expand your chest as you breathe in. Pause for a second or two, then...
5. Breathe out slowly and passively through the mouthpiece until your lungs are completely empty. Let the muscles of your chest and shoulders relax as the air leaves your lungs. Do not force the exhalation.
6. Pause until you feel the urge to breathe in again (approximately one to two seconds).
7. This *fast breath-in, slow breath-out cycle* is considered one repetition. One fast breath in and slow, relaxed breath out will take approximately four to five seconds to complete. If you feel dizzy or light-headed, slow down your breathing, or stop and take a break.
8. Focus on trying to always breathe in as quickly and as deeply as possible, while breathing out as slowly and deeply as possible so that the time between inhalations is long.

The full training routine should be twenty-five repetitions (breaths) twice a day (once in the morning and once in the evening). This adds up to about five minutes of training per day. However, it will take approximately three weeks to work up to the full training routine. Here is a schedule to use.

Week one—Perform ten repetitions twice a day. Week two—Increase to fifteen repetitions twice per day. Week three—Increase to the full training routine of twenty-five repetitions twice per day.

You can increase the resistance by turning the adjustment sleeve clockwise on the BreathBooster®. As you increase the resistance, you will feel a greater tug on your lungs when you draw in through the mouthpiece. Your goal is to set the resistance on your BreathBooster® so that by your last (twenty-fifth) repetition your respiratory muscles are fully fatigued. In other words you are just able to fully complete the twenty-fifth repetition.

Once you are able to complete the full routine of twenty-five repetitions with moderate effort (able to do two or three more repetitions if you had to), increase the resistance for the next training session by turning the sleeve on the training device clockwise one-half to one full rotation.

Remember, if you experience light-headedness, shortness of breath, or a noticeable increase in pulse rate, stop the training session until the symptoms disappear.

If you follow these breathing exercises and the above respiratory training routine, you will be one step closer to healing your damaged cells. Studies and our own clinical experience have shown that increasing blood-oxygen concentration and stimulating the parasympathetic nervous system are crucial factors in managing chronic conditions, including your back pain. These breathing exercises are the easiest, most effective, and least expensive ways to achieve those goals.

So put down the book. Find a quiet place, and get started with the third exercise in this chapter.

CHAPTER 20

ENERGY-RESTORATION DIET

In order to successfully manage back pain, the amount of silent inflammation in the body must be reduced. In addition the body's ability to produce ATP must be improved. One of the most powerful tools to both reduce silent inflammation and boost ATP (energy) production is a proper diet. This chapter describes what this kind of diet looks like, how it curbs silent inflammation, and the reasons why this diet is so important.

Before we get started, we want you to know one very important thing. This is *not* a weight-loss diet. That is why it is named the energy restoration diet. ATP is the sole source of energy for every cell in your body. The sole purpose of this diet is to promote cellular energy and reduce silent inflammation, not to lose weight. We don't want there to be any confusion on this point.

Why worry about cellular energy? A lack of ATP is a major limiting factor for healing damaged tissues. By increasing cellular energy, you better equip the body to heal itself. And as strange as it may sound, your diet can be (and often is) a source of inflammation throughout your body.

Years of diet-related, low-level inflammation can contribute to the chronic stress cycle and to the development of chronic diseases such as spinal decay, peripheral neuropathy, cardiovascular disease, Alzheimer's disease, rheumatoid arthritis, and even certain types of cancer.

Inflammation contributes to these diseases by eliciting an immune-system response and damaging tissues directly, which in turn adds to chronic stress and prevents the natural healing process. What makes diet-related inflammation so damaging is its unique role as both a massive drain on the body's resources (taking energy away from healing and other healthy functions) and its ability to prevent adequate absorption of nutrients from food. You can imagine how dangerous this can be. Silent inflammation is demanding more energy yet limiting the production of energy at the same time.

The energy restoration diet supports recovery in two ways. First, it lowers silent inflammation thus reducing chronic stress and naturally increasing your body's ability to heal. Second, it supports ATP production on a cellular level, so you have more energy to heal damaged nerves. For those reasons we have devoted an especially long chapter to this diet.

This chapter starts off by teaching you why you should be worried about ATP production and silent inflammation. Then you'll learn how certain foods can cause inflammation, followed by a section where we'll examine several gastrointestinal conditions commonly seen in patients. The last and most important part of this chapter will teach you exactly how to implement this diet into your lifestyle.

ATP Production and How It Is Affected by Diet

ATP stands for adenosine triphosphate. It is considered to be the energy currency of life and is the molecule that stores energy to be used by each cell in your body. However, in order to be used as energy, the food we eat must be broken down and then converted to ATP by the body.

We need adequate amounts of ATP just to survive throughout our daily lives. Luckily, there are a number of ways that ATP is made available, and most foods contain the raw materials necessary to create it.

Silent inflammation is a powerful stressor that often uses up too much of the body's supply of energy. Even worse, silent inflammation can actually prevent your body from producing the optimum amount of ATP needed to heal. This is true even if you have reduced your chronic stress using the other therapies of the DICE protocol. If this type of silent inflammation is left unaddressed, it can act as an immense roadblock to healing. In fact people who suffer from less-than-optimum ATP production over long periods of time will almost always develop some sort of disease—a signature of Neuro-Imbalance.

You don't have to understand all the science behind ATP synthesis for this diet to work. Just remember that having enough ATP in your body is critical to almost every cellular process and is one of the keys to managing most chronic diseases, as well as healthy aging.

And modifying your diet just so happens to be the best way to reduce silent inflammation.

SILENT INFLAMMATION

Inflammation is most commonly understood as the redness, tenderness, pain, and swelling that occurs around a cut, scrape, or bruise. Everyone experiences this kind of inflammation, and it is normal. This type of acute (short-term) inflammation is the body's way of healing a damaged area.

The redness and swelling are caused by increased blood flow bringing nutrients to the damaged area. The tenderness and pain are caused by hormones, which lower the pain threshold of the affected area. The pain causes us to guard a wound, protecting it from further damage.

This type of inflammation is healthy; without it we would never recover from wounds or injuries. However, there's another kind of inflammation that occurs in the body that you can't see or feel, but it is destructive and leads to a host of chronic (long-term) diseases…low-level chronic inflammation.

Low-level chronic inflammation is often called silent inflammation. It can occur in any part of the body (brain, joints, arteries, intestines, etc.). It often occurs at such a low level that without very specialized tests, you and your doctor never even realize it is there. Its difficulty to detect resulted in the term *silent inflammation*.

As mentioned earlier silent inflammation is a stressor that uses up large amounts of your energy. It does this by causing the body to tear down more tissues than it rebuilds. Tearing down tissues is a very energy-demanding process. The caveat here is that silent inflammation reduces an affected cell's ability to produce ATP *(Kumar et al. 2005, 4–116)*.

While silent inflammation robs energy from the body, reducing silent inflammation does the opposite. In fact reducing your level of silent inflammation lowers chronic stress giving you more energy to live (and enjoy) life and gives your cells more energy to heal themselves.

Like most stressors, silent inflammation throws off the body's natural hormonal balance. Areas of the body affected by inflammation tell the brain that it is under attack, raising your stress response. This leads to all the typical symptoms of fight-or-flight response including difficulty sleeping, poor short-term memory, and poor blood flow in the extremities.

It just so happens that the typical American diet is one of the biggest causes of silent inflammation and all its chronic-stress-related problems. This does not mean eating the wrong things directly causes your pain, but the silent inflammation caused by the wrong diet *does* prevent countless people from reducing their chronic stress and successfully managing their condition.

How Food Causes Inflammation

There are two main ways food can cause inflammation. The first, and easiest to detect, are allergies and reactivities to specific foods. These are both direct stressors. The second cause of inflammation is when we consume foods that cause the body to release inflammatory hormones. These are indirect stressors. There is a third class of foods you have to watch out for as well. They aren't stressors, and they do not cause inflammation directly, but they do slow down the healing process. For that reason this third group of foods only has to be avoided for a short period of time.

Food Allergies and Reactivities

Foods you are allergic or reactive to may need to be avoided for the rest of your life. When you have an allergy or food reactivity, your body's immune system mistakenly attacks that food causing inflammation in the digestive system and often throughout the whole body. When you eat these kinds of foods, you are not only causing inflammation you are also contributing to chronic stress.

How do people become allergic or reactive to foods? The immune system is designed to keep invaders such as bacteria, viruses, and parasites out of the body. For any number of reasons, a person's immune system can begin to mistake certain foods for foreign invaders. The misidentification of a food item for an invader causes an immune response to that food. Depending on the severity of the response, the action is labeled an allergy or reactivity (also known as an intolerance or sensitivity). The reaction can range from life-threateningly severe to a low-level inflammatory response without noticeable symptoms.

Regardless of the severity of the reaction, any food that causes a damaging immune response creates inflammation in the digestive system and often throughout the entire body.

There are many ways you can become allergic or sensitive to a food. All you need to know is that once it occurs, you have to avoid that food or suffer the consequences: rashes, fatigue, stomach pain, diarrhea, IBS, headaches, itchy mouth, throat, or ears, and, the most insidious of all, silent inflammation.

FOODS THAT PROMOTE INFLAMMATORY HORMONES

There are many foods that, when eaten in the wrong amount or proportion, lead to excess production of inflammatory hormones. The key players in this section are the essential fatty acids (EFAs), sugar, and starch. These foods are not necessarily bad or unhealthy; they just can't be eaten in large quantities or without being balanced by other foods.

For example, consuming high amounts of corn oil can cause problems if it isn't balanced out with enough fish oil. In other words you need to be eating equal amounts of omega-3 and omega-6 fatty acids. (The total amount you eat is much less important than trying to eat equal amounts of each.)

With regards to sugar and starch, you need to ensure that you eat them along with protein and fat, while altogether avoiding simple processed sugars like high-fructose corn syrup (corn syrup), table sugar and refined grain flours which quickly turn into simple sugars, enter the bloodstream, and spike your blood glucose (blood sugar). Take a look at some of the ingredient lists on some foods in your pantry or refrigerator. You'll be shocked at how many packaged foods include these ingredients.

WHY YOU NEED A BALANCE OF OMEGA-3 AND OMEGA-6 FATTY ACIDS

There are two important fatty acids the human body needs and cannot make on its own, hence the name essential fatty acids (EFAs). These EFAs are called omega-3 and omega-6 fatty acids. (You've probably heard of them before.) These EFAs are converted by the body into very important cell-to-cell communication hormones, among other things. Omega-6 fatty acids can be converted into hormones that initiate inflammation, while Omega-3 fatty acids can be turned into hormones that stop inflammation.

What is important to note is that the body functions best when these fatty acids are eaten in equal amounts. Unfortunately, most people eat between ten and twenty times more omega-6 fatty acids than omega-3 fatty acids. This equates to your body initiating more inflammation than you have the ability to stop. The result is a situation where the body breaks tissues down faster than it heals and repairs itself.

This is why a dietary imbalance of omega-3 and omega-6 fatty acids is one of the leading causes of silent inflammation.

How Excess Sugar and Starch Cause Silent Inflammation

Eating carbohydrates causes the body to release a hormone called insulin. Since diabetes is incredibly prevalent in the United States (and is affecting more and more children), you probably already know a thing or two about insulin. But we're going to explain it for those who may not know many details.

To be more accurate, eating both carbohydrates and protein causes the pancreas to release insulin, but carbohydrates cause your pancreas to release much more.

When compared to fat and protein, carbohydrates also cause the body to release smaller amounts of the hormones that make you feel full. In fact fat and certain amino acids (building blocks of proteins) are the only nutrients that stimulate the secretion of cholecystokinin, which tells your brain that you are full *(Sears 2005, 64–5)*. Protein and fat are also superior to carbohydrates because they cause a larger secretion of the "feel full" hormone known as peptide *(Wolf 2010, 62)*.

The lack of the release of the "feel full" hormones, cholecystokinin and peptide YY, when we eat a carb-rich meal can cause us to eat way more carbohydrates (and too much fat and protein as well) than we need. Our digestive tract simply does not receive the "feel full" signal, thus resulting in overeating and excessive insulin release.

So why worry so much about insulin? Insulin is necessary in the right amounts, but it is also an inflammatory hormone by its very nature *(Sears 2005, 210–18; el Boustani et al. 1989, 315–21)*.

When we eat too many carbs, the pancreas releases too much insulin. Over time this results in silent inflammation, insulin resistance, weight gain, even greater insulin resistance, and eventually—for many people—it leads to diabetes.

On the other hand, protein and fat make us feel full quickly and cause the body to release less insulin. But a diet of all fat and protein has its own set of problems. What is the solution? Eat complete meals with the right kinds of protein, carbohydrates, and fat *in the right amount* so that you feel full *before* too much insulin is released. This is how balanced meals prevent silent inflammation.

The key to making the energy-restoration diet work is eating meals that don't leave you feeling hungry. If a meal is balanced, you won't be left hungry. To do this, you need to eat enough fat and protein with every meal.

Aside from promoting overeating and excessive insulin release, carbohydrate-rich meals create another common problem, and the following chain of events usually results: you will overeat, produce too much insulin, and then have a blood glucose drop a few hours later resulting in intense hunger. That situation is never fun; we've all been there. Eating a balanced meal is just as pleasurable as a carbohydrate-heavy one, without the nasty side effects of insulin spikes and crashes, and silent inflammation.

Before we move into the next section, let us introduce you to a concept called glycemic load. As you'll see later on, the energy-restoration diet is all about eating lots of vegetables, fruits, and lean meats. However, fruits and some vegetables (especially starches) can be quite high in carbohydrates and promote an unhealthy jump in blood glucose and insulin, resulting in silent inflammation. One example of a vegetable that has a high glycemic load is potatoes. Many fruits also have high glycemic loads such as bananas, grapes, and raisins.

Glycemic load is a way to calculate how a given serving size of a particular food will affect your blood glucose. Fruits and vegetables whose typical serving size has a high glycemic load are not totally off limits, but they are recommended in smaller serving sizes, and they should never be eaten by themselves. When moderate quantities of carbohydrate-rich foods are combined with fats and proteins, their effect on blood glucose is reduced. This is why eating balanced meals is so important. For example, eating a handful of raisins is bad, while eating the same quantity of a mixture of raisins and nuts is much better.

If you want to know more information about the glycemic load and index, refer to Appendix B in the back of the book.

FOODS THAT PREVENT INTESTINAL HEALING

There is one final category of foods that doesn't cause inflammation directly, but does prevent you from healing, if you are already suffering from gastrointestinal-derived silent inflammation *(Miyake and Tanaka and McNeil 2007, e687)*. These foods only need to be avoided for a short amount of time—while your intestinal barrier is recovering. After that, they can be put back into your regular diet.

These foods include:
- Legumes (beans, peas, and peanuts)
- Nightshade plants (tomatoes, eggplant, and all peppers)
- Alcohol

Nuts, legumes, and nightshade vegetables are healthy and nutritious foods that are not by nature bad for you. They simply slow the healing process for people who are already suffering from silent inflammation, especially for those who suffer from leaky gut syndrome *(Nachbar and Oppenheim 1980, 2338–45)*.

Alcohol is not terrible if consumed in moderation. However, when you are trying to eliminate silent inflammation and boost ATP production, consuming alcohol will slow the process down.

All the foods listed above can be added back into your diet after the initial phase of the energy-restoration diet is complete.

Before we move into the nuts-and-bolts section of the energy-restoration diet, we want to tell you about three more conditions that commonly cause silent inflammation. It has been determined through lab testing that most of our patients suffer from at least one of these conditions. You will probably find yourself saying, "That's exactly what I feel like," or "I had no idea that had anything to do with my pain," so pay close attention. We have made our explanation as brief and nontechnical as possible.

LEAKY GUT, DYSBIOSIS, AND GLUTEN REACTIVITY

Leaky gut syndrome is a term many doctors use for a condition called intestinal permeability. ("Leaky gut" is much easier to say.)

To understand leaky gut, you have to have an idea of what your intestines look like on the inside. So bear with us through this explanation, as it will help you understand much of what is to come in this chapter.

A QUICK LOOK INTO YOUR INTESTINES

The intestines are kind of like a pipe that is lined on the inside with shag carpet. The strings of the shag carpet are where the body absorbs all the nutrients from your food. The strings are called the intestinal villi.

Each string of the carpet (intestinal villi) is covered with hundreds of cells that form a barrier between the mashed up, digesting food inside the intestines and the rest of the body.

These barrier cells (called epithelial cells) act like tollgates for digesting food. Each one of these cellular tollgates monitors what is allowed to pass through the intestinal wall and into the blood stream as well as what is not.

In a healthy person, all nutrients (protein, fat, carbs, and vitamins) pass *through* these cells, never around them. These epithelial tollgates are supposed to hold on tightly to each other so that nothing can squeeze between them and go undetected. Their tightly knit structure forces nutrients to go through the tollgate cells, not around them.

Does this make sense so far? OK, now let's consider a person with leaky gut...

In a person with leaky gut, the tollgate cells (epithelial cells) have gotten so beat up that they can no longer hold onto their neighbors, thus allowing bits of undigested food to squeeze past them. Undigested food can then make it into the bloodstream without passing through the tollgate cells. This is like someone slipping past airport security and getting onto a plane (not a good idea).

If there is one thing the body hates to have in the blood stream, it is food that isn't completely digested. As a result a properly working immune system will mistake undigested food for an invader and wage an all-out war against it. This happens even if it's just some harmless bit of undigested banana.

This war is the normal inflammatory response to keep out invaders, but in this case it's a false alarm. The inflammation only damages the body (since there truly was no invader), and because inflammation is a stressor, it also increases your chronic stress load.

Even worse, after the immune system recognizes a bit of undigested food in the blood stream, it puts the entire immune system on the lookout for that food. In a misdirected effort to be thorough, the immune system throughout the body will now be on the lookout for anything that looks like banana.

If you were in this situation, the next time you took a bite of banana, your immune system would sound the alarm and start attacking the food before it ever made it into the blood stream. If it gets bad enough, your body can even start attacking it from the moment it gets in your mouth. (This extreme reaction is commonly seen in people who develop severe allergies to a food.)

The end result of leaky gut syndrome is massive amounts of inflammation in the intestines. Since undigested food particles are getting through the intestinal barrier, leaky gut almost always leads to inflammation elsewhere in the body. (Wherever those little bits of food wind up, inflammation will follow.) This inflammation will also cause a big increase in your chronic stress load.

The inflammation caused by leaky gut is often silent, meaning you don't need to have stomach problems to have this condition. In reality many patients who never complained of stomachaches or digestive problems were suffering from leaky gut. It wasn't until they were tested that it was apparent that, in order for them to properly heal, they needed to fix their leaky gut first.

What Causes Leaky Gut?

There are many things that can cause leaky gut.
- Chronically high blood glucose
- Chronic stress cycle

- Eating too many grains (especially grains containing gluten) (Drago et al. 2006, 408–19)
- Dysbiosis
- Food allergies
- Infections

As you can see, diet is not the only cause of leaky gut. However, fixing your diet is the *only known* way to successfully manage this condition once you have it. On top of this, if you do in fact have a leaky gut, managing it is crucial to reduce silent inflammation, lower your chronic stress, and regain energy.

You have to realize that a person with leaky gut may never find out exactly what caused it because it is usually the result of several of the above factors. In the end, knowing why you have it is much less important than managing the problem.

Following the energy restoration diet is the only effective way to heal leaky gut, reducing its affect as a stressor and giving your body a chance to heal.

DYSBIOSIS

Dysbiosis is a condition that can occur anywhere in the body where bacteria and fungi are found including the...

- Stomach
- Intestines
- Mouth
- Lungs
- Sinuses
- Surface of the skin

Dysbiosis is an imbalance in the microbiome of a particular place in or on the body. We will focus on the digestive tract since it is the most common place for dysbiosis to occur. The microbiome of the intestines refers to the hundreds of types of bacteria and fungi that normally occur in your intestines.

Certain bacteria and fungi are supposed to be in your intestines. (They aid in digestion and other metabolic processes.) There are also bacteria, fungi, and parasites that aren't supposed to be there. (They cause problems like diarrhea, bloating, and—in extreme cases—life-threatening infections.)

If your intestines have a large amount of a bacteria or a fungus that isn't supposed to be there, you have an infection. If you have more bad bacteria than normal, but not enough to cause pain and major discomfort, you may be in an in-between state called dysbiosis.

This in-between state means you have enough bad bacteria, fungi, or parasites to cause health problems but not enough to cause the pain, noticeable inflammation, or fever that a doctor can easily diagnose as an infection. Its lack of clear symptoms is why dysbiosis is rarely diagnosed.

WHAT CAUSES DYSBIOSIS

Dysbiosis can often be attributed to antibiotic use *(Quévrain and Seksik 2013, 45–51)*. Antibiotics don't just target bad bacteria; most are designed to kill any bacteria (whether good or bad). This is a problem since the good bacteria in your intestines play a very important role in your health. Killing off the good bacteria turns your intestines into unclaimed land that can be overtaken by bad bacteria once you finish the antibiotic.

However, recent research suggests that poor diet alone can be a major contributor to dysbiosis. In fact eating a poor diet for as little as one day can cause a noticeable change in the microbiome of the small intestines *(Turnbaugh et al. 2009, 6ra14).*

Dysbiosis can also be caused by long-term antacid use or the use of other medications that lower the acidity of your stomach. The acid in your stomach has the extremely important job of killing off most bacteria found on food. (This is a good thing.)

Overt-the-counter antacids, and many prescription heartburn medications, reduce the acidity of your stomach. This, in turn, allows bacteria to survive the trip through your stomach and to make their way into your intestines where they can live and reproduce, causing all sorts of problems including silent inflammation.

What Dysbiosis Does to Your Body

An imbalance in your intestinal microbiome can hurt you in three ways. First and foremost, the intestinal microbiota has an important role in immune system function. Second, the byproducts produced by excessive amounts of certain intestinal microorganisms can be toxic *(Brown et al. 2012, 1095–1119).* These toxins are called endotoxins, and they act as a stressor. Endotoxins can over time begin to irritate the lining of the intestines. This irritation can lead to leaky gut syndrome, another major stressor, as you now know.

Aside from leaky gut, dysbiosis can cause silent inflammation *(Anders and Andersen and Stecher 2013; Aleshukina 2012, 74–8),* irritable bowel syndrome *(DuPont and DuPont 2011, 523–31),* gas, bloating, indigestion, bad breath, diarrhea, constipation, fatigue, and can contribute to various other diseases and symptoms.

How to Fix Dysbiosis

The good news is dysbiosis can be reversed. In the short term it can be easily eliminated using antibiotics. But if you remember from above, antibiotics are often the causes of dysbiosis in the first place. Antibiotics often get rid of the dysbiosis for a week or two, but the bad bacteria move right back in if nothing else is changed, and this time with less competition from good bacteria.

A better way to get rid of dysbiosis is to go on the energy restoration diet. By doing so, you will reduce the amount of simple sugars in your diet (the primary food of bad bacteria). We also recommend that you take probiotic supplements that will help colonize the good bacteria to fight off the bad bacteria *(Walker and Lawley 2013, 75–86)*.

As a long-term solution, eating unpasteurized, fermented foods like sauerkraut, pickles, and others on a regular basis will provide you with a natural supply of probiotics.

Dysbiosis in a Nutshell

Dysbiosis is an imbalance between the good and bad bacteria in the intestines. When it occurs it can lead to many intestinal problems as well as health problems throughout the body.

Dysbiosis has many causes including antibiotic use and antacid use. Luckily, fixing dysbiosis can be as simple as modifying your diet and taking a probiotic supplement.

GLUTEN REACTIVITY

Gluten is a protein found in wheat, barley, rye, and other related grains. Gluten reactivity is one of the most serious health threats of our time. To make matters worse, food manufacturers and the media have latched onto gluten-free diets to get attention and sell products, turning gluten free into a fad diet.

The recent media attention that has been given to gluten-free diets is a double-edged sword. It has increased awareness about a serious health issue, but it has made many people very skeptical of its legitimacy. We are always skeptical of any new health fad, and you should be too.

However, gluten *reactivity* is not a fad. It is an inflammatory cascade that occurs in a startling number of people. It is especially common in people with neurological conditions, chronic low energy, Alzheimer's disease, gastrointestinal problems (like IBS, acid reflux, chronic indigestion, etc.), autoimmune diseases, and many other conditions that seem totally unrelated to eating gluten-containing foods.

Gluten reactivity is not a classic allergy. That's why it's so difficult to diagnose. The standard tests doctors use to find out what you are allergic to won't tell them whether or not you are reactive to gluten. The gluten reactivity test is a much newer and more sensitive test. Even the more in-depth biopsy test used to diagnose celiac disease (an extreme form of gluten reactivity) won't always tell you if you are reactive to gluten.

Although gluten reactivity is not a classic allergy (although for many people it will progress to that), it is still a serious medical condition. The fact that gluten reactivity is not a classic allergy may be its most dangerous characteristic. Gluten reactivity is rarely diagnosed unless it leads to celiac disease.

The result?

Tens of thousands of people suffer from this disorder without knowing it. To make matters worse, undiagnosed gluten reactivity or celiac disease acts as a stressor adding to chronic stress, and often contributes to chronic diseases such as Alzheimer's disease, various autoimmune disorders, peripheral neuropathy, and others.

HOW CAN WHEAT POSSIBLY BE BAD FOR ME?

For many years we have been told that whole wheat is a wonder food. For those who are gluten reactive and for those with celiac disease, eating wheat (even whole wheat) can cause serious health problems including intestinal permeability (leaky gut), autoimmune diseases *(Eisenmann et al. 2009, 168–71)*, and neurological disorders *(Hadjivassiliou et al. 2006, 1262–6; Ludvigsson et al. 2007, 1317–27)*. As you already know, leaky gut can lead to many chronic disorders throughout the body.

Here's how it works. If you are gluten reactive, the gluten protein fools your body into thinking that gluten is invading bacteria. Your body responds by transporting undigested gluten into your intestinal walls so that your immune system can ambush it. This is a very sneaky trick your body plays on invaders. Once the suspicious particle is inside the intestinal walls, the immune system destroys and digests it.

When your immune system does this to bacteria, it is saving you from an infection. When it does this little immune-system trick on gluten, it wastes and diverts your body's valuable energy. Attacking gluten also causes inflammation and damage in the area where the ambush took place. Your body's immune system takes a scorched earth approach to killing invaders. This means some of your body's healthy cells will be damaged in the crossfire. As resilient as the body typically is, it cannot replace the healthy cells as quickly as they are being destroyed.

Remember, small amount of damage done to your body during an immune response is completely normal. Attacking a few bacteria or viruses here and there is no big deal. Your body quickly repairs itself, and all is well.

However, when a gluten-reactive person eats a slice of bread or some pasta, the body is required to attack thousands of gluten proteins throughout the intestines all at once.

Now imagine this same scenario happening over and over again to someone, due to habits of consistently eating products containing gluten (or any other reactive food source for that matter). It doesn't look pretty, does it? Eventually this immune response leads to leaky gut.

How?

People who are gluten reactive have generally eaten gluten repeatedly, often at every meal, for a long time. Their intestines become so depleted and chronically inflamed that they can no longer close up the space between the epithelial cells in the microvilli of the intestines. This is a textbook case of leaky gut. Once you have developed leaky gut syndrome, larger molecules and bacteria can get inside your body and cause even more inflammation.

As this process continues, your body will do one or more of the following things.

1) You may develop allergies to many foods because they are able to pass through the intestinal walls and into the blood stream undigested.

2) Your body may develop antibodies to your own tissues. (This is called autoimmunity.) Your immune system may now start attacking various tissues throughout the body. These tissues may include muscle fibers (causing muscle pain anywhere

in the body), nerve cells (causing neuropathies) *(Alaedini et al. 2007, 6590–5)*, or joint tissues (causing arthritis).

3) The inflammation that occurs causes an enormous amount of stress on your body. This stress adds to the chronic stress cycle causing your body to do several things, including the following.

- Deplete its energy supplies
- Reduce circulation to the hands and feet
- Make sleeping difficult
- Cause poor short-term memory
- Cause further digestive upsets

Being reactive to gluten does not mean that you will experience all of these problems. However, if you are reactive to gluten, you will have problems somewhere, even if you don't notice anything yet. Damage is being done.

We must be clear. We're not suggesting that everyone is gluten reactive, nor do we believe that a gluten-free diet is the secret to curing everyone's conditions. But it is way more prevalent than we are led to believe.

Removing gluten is often the critical step that takes patients from feeling "a little bit better" to "Wow, Doc! I actually slept a whole night without pain."

As with any diet, a few unconvinced patients (who tested gluten positive) think it's OK to cheat a little. Eventually, though, they learn how important it is to go completely off gluten to feel better. Oftentimes patients get frustrated after a few weeks of treatment without seeing the results they want. When they talk to our other gluten-reactive patients, they discover that most of the other patients are seeing great results after having made the lifestyle change.

When these formerly unconvinced patients finally cut out gluten for just a few weeks, they start seeing results. That's usually when they admit they weren't following the diet.

The moral of the story is that cheating on this diet only hurts you. On a normal diet, you can cheat a couple times a week and still lose weight. A gluten-free diet is completely different. (Remember it's not about weight loss at all.) If you test gluten positive, you are either all in or all out. You can't just cut back a little on gluten and get results.

At the risk of sounding like a broken record, we're going to repeat this one more time. If you are gluten reactive, you will only notice a difference if you go completely gluten free.

At this point you may be a little confused about the difference between the energy-restoration diet and a gluten-free diet. Everyone who uses the energy-restoration diet will be gluten free for a certain amount of time regardless of any gluten test results. The difference is that those who are not reactive to gluten can eventually reintroduce it into their diets in small amounts after the initial phase, while those who *are* gluten sensitive must remain gluten free forever.

How the Energy-Restoration Diet Works

There are three phases of the energy-restoration diet. Before going any further, we want to reemphasize the fact that this is not a weight-loss diet or a calorie-restrictive diet. You never need to allow yourself to get hungry on this diet.

Phase one is the most restrictive. During this time you'll be whipping your digestive tract back into shape. This phase reduces your level of silent inflammation, enables your body to produce more ATP, and initiates the healing.

Phase two slowly reintroduces several of the foods you avoided during the first phase. However, this phase still eliminates several of the most commonly inflammatory foods to allow your body to continue healing.

Phase three is when more of the foods you had previously cut out of your diet can be added back in. Reintroducing them slowly gives you a chance to see how your body reacts.

The final phase is the maintenance phase. The goal here is to maintain a healthy, balanced diet. It is more of a lifestyle than a diet. We recommend staying on the maintenance phase of the energy-restoration diet for the rest of your life. It helps you maintain high levels of energy and low levels of inflammation without permanently depriving you of your comfort foods.

Forever seems like a long time when you are talking about diets. We understand. We have all have been on the maintenance phase of the energy diet since 2011, and we're also gluten- and dairy-free. The good news is that you will feel so much better at the end of phase three that you probably won't want to go back.

We simply tell our patients to complete the first three phases to see how much better they feel, then make the decision on whether to make the maintenance phase a permanent lifestyle.

Believe it not, 90 percent of our patients stay on the maintenance phase without us saying much of anything. These people feel so much better that you couldn't talk them into going back.

Enough of all the background information, let's dig into the details of the energy-restoration diet.

PHASE ONE

This phase of the diet only lasts thirty days. For sufferers with severe digestive problems, we typically suggest sixty days.

During this time you will only be eating fruits, vegetables, and meats. The following foods will be off limits:

- All grains and flours—wheat, corn, oats, rice, millet, sorghum, tapioca, buckwheat, etc.
- Dairy—milk, cheese, butter, yogurt, most margarines, and most shortenings
- Legumes—beans, soy, peas, or peanuts
- Highly processed packaged foods
- Refined sugars—table sugar, high-fructose corn syrup, or corn sugar
- Artificial sweeteners: Sweet'N Low, Equal, etc. (These are neurotoxins.)
- MSG—monosodium glutamate
- Alcohol
- Nightshade vegetables—tomatoes, peppers, eggplant, and potatoes

Don't worry. There are a lot of foods you can still eat. It is much easier to focus on what you *can* eat rather than what you cannot. When you are on this diet, you can eat nearly any meat product, fruit, or vegetable you want. When you think of it as a meat, vegetable, and fruit diet, it doesn't seem all that hard.

Just to make it easier on you, we've compiled a list of items you can and can't eat for this phase of the diet. You can find the list in the back of this book in Appendix A.

While on this diet, you will need to buy more minimally processed foods and fresh foods to avoid things like wheat and dairy products. To make this easier, shop the perimeter of the grocery store, and avoid straying into the center aisles too often. Fresh veggies, fruits, meats, and eggs are almost always along the outside walls of the store. Staying out of the center aisles makes it much easier to avoid temptation.

In addition to using the list in Appendix A, you will need to get into the habit of thoroughly checking labels for ingredients. You will be shocked at how many food items use wheat, dairy, and soy as cheap fillers.

Once the thirty days are up, you move right into phase two.

PHASE TWO

This phase lasts thirty days as well. During phase two, you will be able to reintroduce several items that you cut out during phase one. You will need to reintroduce these items one at a time. We recommend adding one or two new items per week. This gives you a chance to see how you feel when you eat each food and notice if you have any reactions. Because of this process of gradually adding back in foods, this kind of diet is often called an elimination and challenge diet. This reintroduction process is critical if you want to find out what foods, if any, you are reactive to. (It might not be the item you suspect.)

Here are some common reactions to look for.

- Headache
- Digestive upsets
- Skin rashes or irritation
- Itching scalp or skin
- Mouth sores
- Itching mouth or throat
- Lack of energy
- Fatigue
- Brain fog (loss of mental sharpness or trouble focusing)
- Back pain
- Flare-up of your primary symptoms

If you notice any of those symptoms, stop eating that food item immediately. Then try to eat it again in a week. If, after a week's interval, you experience the same reaction again, you are likely reactive to that food. You should avoid that food for the entire duration of the first three phases of the energy-restoration diet. You may test that food again (once you are in the maintenance phase) just to be sure.

During phase two you can reintroduce the following foods.

- Most *gluten-free* grains—rice, millet, quinoa, buckwheat, tapioca (no corn)
- Legumes—but no soy products
- Most nightshade vegetables—bell peppers, peppers, eggplant, potatoes, but *tomatoes are still off limits*

Remember to reintroduce these items to your diet one item at a time. It may take longer than thirty days before you have reintroduced all the foods. That's fine. Start by reintroducing the ones you most enjoy; you can reintroduce the others later.

The following foods are *still off limits* for phase two of the energy-restoration diet.

- Gluten-containing grains: wheat, barley, rye, oats, etc.
- Corn
- Alcohol
- Soy products—soy beans, oil, tofu, soy milk
- Dairy products
- Tomato products—sauces, ketchup, tomato-based salsa, etc.
- Refined sugars

Once you have completed thirty days of phase two, you can move into phase three.

PHASE THREE

During the third phase of the diet, you will continue to reintroduce all nightshades (including tomatoes), legumes (except soy), gluten-free grains, and sugar (in limited amounts).

Once again, eat only one or two new food items per week. You still need to challenge your body with a couple new food items per week to see if you have any reactions. This is a common, no-cost way to test for food allergies and reactivities.

The only restrictions for phase three are the following.

- No gluten-containing grains (wheat, barley, rye, and oats)
- No dairy
- No soy

This phase of the diet also lasts for thirty days.

PHASE FOUR

Phase four is the maintenance phase of the energy diet. There are fewer restrictions for this phase. It is designed to promote a flexible dietary plan that you can stick with for the long haul. The goal here is to provide you with the maximum amount of health benefits with a minimum amount of dietary restriction.

If you have been tested for gluten or dairy reactivity, and the tests came back negative (no gluten or dairy sensitivity), you can start to reintroduce these foods into your diet.

However, you should not start eating gluten and dairy foods on a regular basis. Make them an occasional treat. You may not be reactive to them, but they still limit overall energy, play games with your blood glucose, and increase silent inflammation throughout your body.

Structure your daily diet so that you limit these indulgences to the weekends or special occasions. By limiting them you can still enjoy these foods guilt free, while keeping your energy levels up and silent inflammation low. As with any diet plan, it must be livable, or you won't stay on it.

Regardless of any food sensitivity, you will want to continue to limit your intake of the following items.

- Refined sugars—sugar, cane sugar, beet sugar, corn sugar, corn syrup, high-fructose corn syrup, dextrose, etc.
- Artificial sweeteners—Avoid these; they are neurotoxins (kill your precious neurons).
- MSG—monosodium glutamate (also a neurotoxin)
- Gluten-containing grains—wheat, barley, rye, etc.
- Dairy products (all milk/cream/cheese that comes from an animal)
- Soy products—You can eat soy lecithin, a common food emulsifier.

Those who are gluten or diary reactive need to permanently remove these items from their diet. Nearly everyone who is gluten or dairy reactive will occasionally splurge and eat the food they are reactive to. This is not a sin; don't beat yourself up over it or feel guilty. That will only increase your stress response.

If you are going to eat something you are reactive to, enjoy it, and get back on the wagon ASAP. You will most likely suffer some digestive discomfort or other symptoms later on. Because of these negative consequences, your desire to splurge will most likely diminish as you get used to your new lifestyle and realize how great you feel when you avoid those foods.

A special note about oats...

While oats do not naturally contain gluten, almost all oats are harvested, transported, and processed with equipment used for wheat. Due to this cross contamination, they will usually cause problems for those who are gluten reactive. There are certain brands of oats that are certified gluten free and are processed in dedicated wheat-free facilities. These brands are usually trustworthy, but you must be careful. Test these products in small amounts, and make your own decision.

BUILDING A BALANCED, HIGH-ENERGY MEAL

Thus far you've learned a lot about diet, but we haven't mentioned any guidelines for how much of each kind of food you should be eating. As promised early on, there are no points and no weighing out portions. We like to keep it simple. The easiest way to build a balanced meal is to divide your plate into thirds and then fill one-third with lean proteins (lean meats) and the other two-thirds with vegetables. If you are going to eat fruit with a meal, it should be in a small quantity along with a larger quantity of low glycemic load (nonstarchy) vegetables. If you plan on having a meal with fruit and protein only, the portion of fruit should be small.

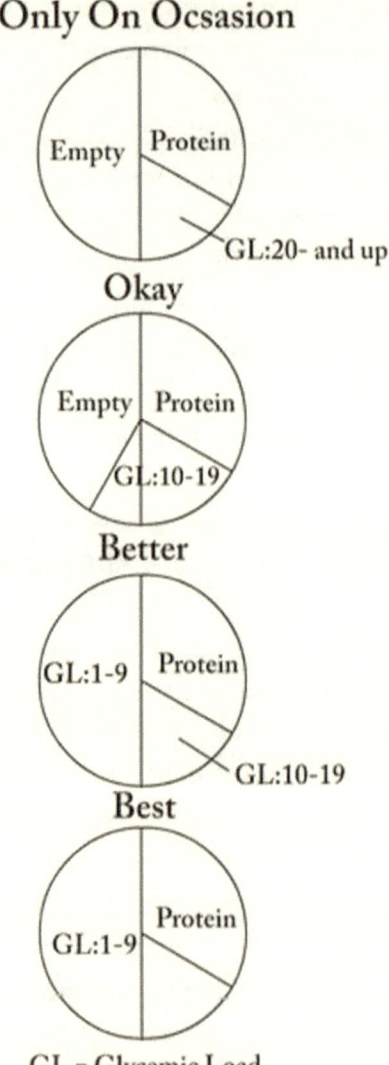

GL = Glycemic Load

Meal building using Glycemic Load: How your plate should look if
you are building a low-inflammation high-energy meal.

The previous diagram shows you how these three general
meal types should look. As you can see, this system is very

flexible, but you must keep in mind that the vegetable-and-protein-only option is the best for low inflammation and high energy. An additional consideration is the glycemic load of the vegetable or fruit you are planning on eating. For example, if you are in phase four of the diet—where potatoes are allowed—and you decide to eat a potato dish, you should consider them as a fruit not a vegetable. Their glycemic load is more similar to fruit than most other vegetables. For that reason your portion of potatoes should be quite small and accompanied with other low-glycemic vegetables. Also, soluble fiber slows the absorption of glucose from fruits and vegetables, so you should choose foods high in soluble fiber to keep you blood glucose levels in line *(Sears 2005, 51).*

This basic guide should ensure that your meals are well balanced, make you feel full quickly, keep your energy levels high, and keep silent inflammation at bay.

THIS DIET IS EASY

It's true. You may have been surprised at how brief the how-to section of the energy-restoration diet was. The theory behind this diet may be complex, but the diet itself is pretty simple. There are no calories to count, no points to add up, no miracle pills, and no monthly fees. There aren't any gimmicks either. You don't have to weigh out portions or order frozen meals. After the initial adjustment, most people find this diet easy to stick with (especially since they usually feel a whole lot better).

Unlike most weight loss diets, which leave you hungry, cranky, and feeling puny, the energy-restoration diet actually makes you feel better.

CHEATING

There is always a temptation to cheat on a diet. Removing foods that you may love is never easy. However, unlike most diets where the goal is losing weight, this diet completely relies on you not cheating in order for it to work.

If you cheat during the first ninety days of the diet, you will lose many of the benefits. For the first ninety days, it's an all-or-nothing affair. You have to be totally committed in order to see most of the life-changing results. Don't torture yourself by committing half way. You will be depriving yourself with very little benefit.

SUPER FOODS AND SPICES

There are hundreds of foods out there that are packed full of protective nutrients and have anti-inflammatory or energy-boosting properties. These "super foods" should be incorporated into your new lifestyle as much as possible.

The following list will get you familiar with some of the most common super foods and spices. Make eating a few of them each day a priority.

- Cruciferous vegetables—cabbages, broccoli, cauliflower, brussels sprouts, collard greens, arugula, radishes, turnips, kale, watercress, and mustard greens
- Dark berries—blueberries, blackberries, boysenberries, raspberries, strawberries, etc.
- Dark grapes
- Colorful fruits—Make sure you eat a good variety of colors. Different colors correspond to different antioxidants.

- Coconut
- Coconut oil
- Olives
- Extra-virgin olive oil
- Ginger root—as a spice or as a tea
- Rosemary—as a spice
- Turmeric—Combine it with black pepper for maximum absorption.

The foods mentioned above are some of the best super foods, but there are dozens more. In general most spices are very healthy. The energy-restoration diet will encourage you to cook differently, so it is a great time to learn to incorporate new spices into your cooking.

Learning to cook with new spices is also a great way to avoid dwelling on what you can't have. There are so many flavors and combinations of spices to be explored. If you focus on these new flavors and foods, this diet will be much more enjoyable. Who knows? You may find foods you love even more than the ones you had to give up.

A Word on Artificial Sweeteners and Other Food Additives

Artificial sweeteners can be very confusing. Some studies say they are fine while others say they contribute to your risk of cancer and other diseases. Instead of offering bulletproof evidence for or against artificial sweeteners, we can offer you this test in common sense.

The studies that show artificial sweeteners to be a healthy sugar alternative are funded by the same companies that produce them. These companies stand to lose a lot of money if these sweeteners are found to be dangerous. In contrast the studies that suggest that these sweeteners could pose long-term health risks were largely funded by independent groups with very little to gain other than knowledge.

It's pretty clear to us that there was some bias going on in the studies funded by sweetener producers. We highly discourage people from using artificial sweeteners. In fact we would rather see our patients use real sugar than artificial sweeteners.

Many of our patients have had very obvious negative reactions to artificial sweeteners once they were reintroduced (after avoiding them for several months).

RECOMMENDED ALTERNATIVE SWEETENER

One sweetener that works well, and that we highly recommend, is Stevia. It is a natural, plant-based sweetener. Stevia has been used in Japan as the main sugar substitute since the 1970s and has been available in the United States since the mid 1990s. There are no known health risks of using Stevia, and it does not raise blood glucose levels (great for diabetics).

We also find that honey or agave nectar is a great alternative to table sugar or syrup and works great for baking.

MSG

Another common food additive to watch out for is MSG (monosodium glutamate). MSG is a flavor enhancer that, like salt, brings out the flavor in food. It was developed as a way to enhance the flavor of food without adding more salt (so food can be advertised as low sodium).

Studies on MSG are similar to those on artificial sweeteners. The studies funded by the food industry show it is not dangerous, and those performed by outside, independent groups show many potentially dangerous consequences. In several laboratory studies by major universities, rats fed MSG suffered from serious neurological damage *(Gonzalex-Burgos and Perez-Vega and Beas-Zarate 2001, 69–72; Seress et al. 1984, 453–7)*. This makes some sense because glutamate, a component of MSG, is a well-known excitoxin *(Manev et al. 1989, 106–12)*.

When neurons become overexcited, they can cause damage and even cell death. There is no question; glutamate in the wrong amount is a neurotoxin. If you are suffering from any chronic condition, there's no good reason why you should be ingesting any amount of a known neurotoxin if it can be avoided. That being said, we highly recommend permanently removing artificial sweeteners and MSG from your diet. And it is absolutely crucial that you completely remove these items for at least the first ninety days of the energy-restoration diet.

THE ENERGY-RESTORATION DIET, BLOOD GLUCOSE REGULATION, AND FAT METABOLISM

The energy-restoration diet was not specifically designed for diabetics, but in our experience it is the best diet for blood-glucose regulation. Here's why.

The highest glycemic (blood-glucose raising) foods are eliminated, and most importantly, grains (especially wheat) and refined sugars are mostly, if not totally, eliminated. Believe it or not, an ounce of white bread raises your blood glucose just as much as an ounce of table sugar. That's why bread, pasta, and breaded food are just as bad for diabetics as foods with lots of added sugar.

Oftentimes, simply eliminating grains and sugar is enough to give you much more control over your blood glucose. If you follow the above guidelines for eating a well-rounded meal of protein, fat, and good carbohydrates, you will be doing even better. Eating a well-balanced meal limits the spike in your blood glucose after eating.

If you are really serious about getting control over your blood glucose, you should become familiar with the glycemic load of foods you eat.

It just so happens that weight loss is another great side benefit of lowering the amount of insulin your body releases after each meal. Many people don't realize it, but insulin is the primary hormone responsible for fat storage. When you eat too much sugar, or eat foods like wheat and other grains that are easily converted into glucose and absorbed into the blood stream, your body responds by releasing large amounts of insulin. This large amount of insulin tells the cells of your body to absorb glucose (sugar) from the blood for storage. Much of that excess glucose is stored as fat.

In contrast a meal rich in protein and good fats, along with moderate amounts of carbohydrates, stimulates the release of just the right amount of insulin, along with the release of glucagon (insulin's counterpart), which causes a steady release of glucose into the blood stream to feed your body's glucose needs.

By following this particular diet, you will avoid the energy rush and crash that typically follows a carb-heavy meal and, instead, have a steady amount of energy until your next snack or meal.

To sum it up, you need to eat meals with the right balance of protein, fat, and carbohydrates. Limiting high-glycemic foods (like grains and processed sugar) will give you better control over your blood glucose. This diet will also dramatically boost your energy levels and aid in any weight loss you may be looking for. Many of our patients find that this diet has helped them regain the energy of their younger years, which serves as yet another side benefit of the energy-restoration diet.

BREAKFAST, THE MOST IMPORTANT MEAL OF THE DAY

This old saying has much truth to it—especially for those who want to feel great, have high energy all day, and avoid midmorning or afternoon energy crashes. This section explains how breakfast can set your daily hormones and energy level off on the right track.

Breakfast is literally the meal that breaks your fast. It's the first meal you eat after fasting for eight to ten hours. Remember, every time you go to sleep at night, your body is entering a fasting state.

For most of us, fasting throughout the night is not a problem. If you have eaten appropriately throughout the day, and especially in the evening, you should have no problem fasting until morning.

How you break the nighttime fast will affect your energy, hormones, and hunger patterns for the rest of the day.

The secret is to have a breakfast that is high in protein along with some fat and carbohydrates. If you remember from earlier, fat and protein stimulate the release of glucose into the blood stream.

This is exactly what you need to get your motor running in the morning. You want just enough glucose in the blood stream for all your daily activities but not so much that your body releases too much insulin (which pulls the glucose out of the blood stream). Striking this balance is best done with a high-protein breakfast accompanied with good fats and slow-release carbohydrates.

If a low-carb breakfast is good, is a *no*-carb breakfast better? No. If you eat nothing but protein and fat, you will be releasing stored glucose without replacing what you are using. Having a small amount of carbohydrates is important. For example, a breakfast of two eggs alone is OK. Throw in some mixed vegetables or a small wedge of cantaloupe, and it becomes a whole lot better.

If you do the opposite, eat a lot of carbs and less protein, you will get a quick burst of energy from all the glucose followed by an evening crash. A good example of this would be having a bagel and coffee for breakfast. Again, it's all about striking a balance.

How does your breakfast affect your whole day? When your blood glucose crashes from eating a carb-heavy meal, you will naturally crave sugar. Fulfilling those sugar cravings sets up another energy spike and crash. If you eat a good breakfast, you won't crave the foods that cause an energy crash later in the day. As a result your next snack or meal is more likely to be well balanced.

In fact a study conducted by the University of Texas in El Paso demonstrated that increasing the amount of calories eaten at breakfast reduces the total number of calories eaten in a day!

Here's the theory behind this counterintuitive finding. If you eat a bad breakfast or no breakfast, you will usually have a midmorning crash. When you feel the crash, you are more likely to eat a bad snack or drink a caffeinated beverage such as coffee or a diet soda. Once the sugar rush from the snack and caffeine (caffeine raises blood glucose) wears off, you will crash just in time for lunch. Because the crash has left your blood glucose very low, you will once again crave sugar.

These cravings cause you to eat a carb-heavy lunch, setting you up for another crash in the midafternoon. This pattern usually continues all day.

If you are like most people, you've spent years on this blood-glucose roller coaster fueled by high glycemic foods and unbalanced meals. Your energy levels feel like a yo-yo, and you don't know what's wrong. Most people live this way, but you don't have to. By incorporating a good breakfast into the energy-restoration diet, you can smooth out your energy levels so you rarely feel crashes and maintain a constant, steady level of high energy throughout the day.

EXAMPLES OF HIGH-ENERGY BREAKFAST OPTIONS:

Traditional Breakfast One
- Eggs (one to four)
- One-half orange or grapefruit
- Traditional Breakfast Two
- Low-sodium bacon (two to four slices) or ham (a piece the size of your palm)
- Mixed fruit (one-half to one cup of grapes, apple, pineapple, melon)
- Nontraditional option
- Chicken (a piece the size of your palm)—Cold, precooked chicken is a quick, easy breakfast source of protein and fat.

- Steamed vegetables—If you want to use veggies as a source of carbs, be sure to include carrots or some other vegetable that has some sugar in it; a cup of broccoli won't give you the carbs you need.

These are just three quick examples of how to build a complete high-energy breakfast. Be creative, and include foods you love even if they aren't traditionally considered breakfast foods.

SNACKING

Snacking is not only allowed on the energy-restoration diet, it's highly recommended. The trick is to snack right. A good snack requires the same balance as any good meal. It needs to contain protein, fat, and carbs.

A snack of just carbs, even if it sounds healthy (like dried fruit or an apple), can cause you to crash or to get hungry again an hour later. To feel full you must eat some protein or fat.

Snacks usually need to be quick, easy, and portable. Nuts are a great source of protein and fat for snacks. They can be mixed with raisins or other dried fruits and taken just about anywhere. (Just make sure there are more nuts than fruit.) You can also get a quick protein snack from beef jerky. (Make sure it doesn't contain soy sauce, caramel color, malt flavoring, or other sources of gluten.)

Another snack option is to simply eat a few bites of leftover meat along with half an avocado, some olives, or a small piece of fruit.

DINING OUT

In the early phases of the program, it will be very difficult to eat at a restaurant due to so many common foods being restricted. However, in phases three and in the maintenance phase you will want to eat out with friends and family. This can be risky if you are gluten or dairy sensitive, but there are several steps you can take to reduce your risk of getting contaminated (receiving an accidental amount of the allergen in a food that you didn't suspect would contain it.)

Stick to the basics when you eat out. You should choose simple dishes that contain only a few ingredients. For example, a steak and baked potato with steamed veggies or a side salad has very little risk of containing wheat or dairy.

Just be sure to tell the waiter or waitress ahead of time that you do not want butter on the potato and that you need veggies grilled in oil instead of butter (if you are not getting them steamed). In addition make sure there isn't cheese or croutons on the salad.

Avoid dishes that have creamy sauces, since they usually contain wheat flour, dairy, or both.

Salads entrées are another great option because they usually list all of their ingredients (and things can easily be left out). Be sure to ask what's in the dressing. If they don't know the ingredients, ask for olive oil and vinegar.

Luckily, many restaurants are starting to offer gluten-free options. This makes eating out very easy and stress free.

Use This Diet as a Secret Weapon

Once you have completed the first ninety days of the diet, you will officially be on the maintenance phase.

The maintenance phase is your new lifestyle. It should allow you to occasionally indulge in treats. However, many people go back to the stricter phase one part of the diet for a few days when they have overindulged or feel their energy levels dropping. This quickly strategy gets them feeling great again.

Remember, you can always revisit any phase of the diet. Simply follow the instructions for that section for as long as you want. Some people use phase one for just a few days (especially if they accidentally eat some wheat or dairy), others revisit phase one for several weeks each year.

Think of phases one and two as tools you can use to feel better. Once you have completed all three phases (ninety days) feel free to use them how you see fit. You will get a feel for what works for you.

CHAPTER 21

EXERCISE–HOW TO STICK WITH IT

"Feel Good to Exercise" Versus "Putting the Cart before the Horse"

"**E**xercise to feel good" is a concept that has been continuously ingrained into our brains. In order to feel good and become healthy, we need to exercise. It is not a wrong idea. It just isn't entirely correct either. The fact is that many people do not have the energy to start or maintain an exercise program due to being in the chronic stress cycle.

Think about it. If we all know exercise is good for us, then why are we not all signing up for gym memberships and following through with them? Or why are we no longer able to play with grandchildren, go to sporting events, engage in outside activities, etc.? If time isn't your excuse, what is?

Most likely you do not have the energy, or you are afraid of causing further pain or harm. And who could blame you? After knowing what you know now, how could you simply jump into the gym expecting to attain this facade of health without having your body's full support?

This is why we are shifting that thought pattern from exercising first and then feeling good to "feel good to exercise." Just as you can't pull the cart without the horse (your horse is your body), without your body being Neuromechanically Balanced, you are essentially jumping ahead of yourself or "putting the cart before the horse." Your body will be able to promote and express health once you have decreased your chronic stress load. Better yet, once you are Neuromechanically Balanced, you will feel like exercising. Doesn't that sound great?

WHAT IS YOUR CORE, AND HOW DO YOU TRAIN IT?

Interestingly enough, society has recognized this low back pain epidemic and has emphasized the importance of exercising your core muscles.

But what are core muscles?

The core is comprised of a number of muscles that work together to achieve and maintain a stable spine. A stable and strong core is what allows us to successfully move our hips, legs, and arms without injury. Contrary to popular belief, your core muscles are those that make up the front in addition to those in the back. Too many people spend large amounts of time working on only one part of their core by doing countless sit-ups and wonder why they're not getting the anticipated results. They are forgetting about the back musculature! (As you now know, diet is also an integral piece of the puzzle to achieving wellness.)

The core back musculature are the small, deep stability muscles known as multifidi (remember these?), rotatores, and intertransversarii while the erector spinae group, quadratus lumborum, latissimus dorsi, and thoracolumbar fascia are the larger movement muscles (or fascia) of the back. In the front are your deep abdominal muscles, known as internal and external obliques and transverse abdominis, and the most superficial (closest to surface) is the rectus abdominis (the *six-pack*). Together these make up your midsection that everyone refers to as your core

Back Core Musculature

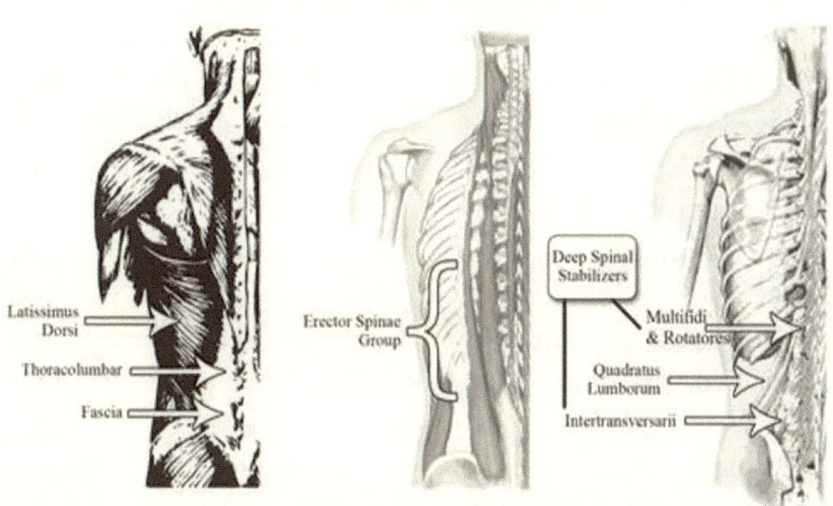

Front Core Musculature

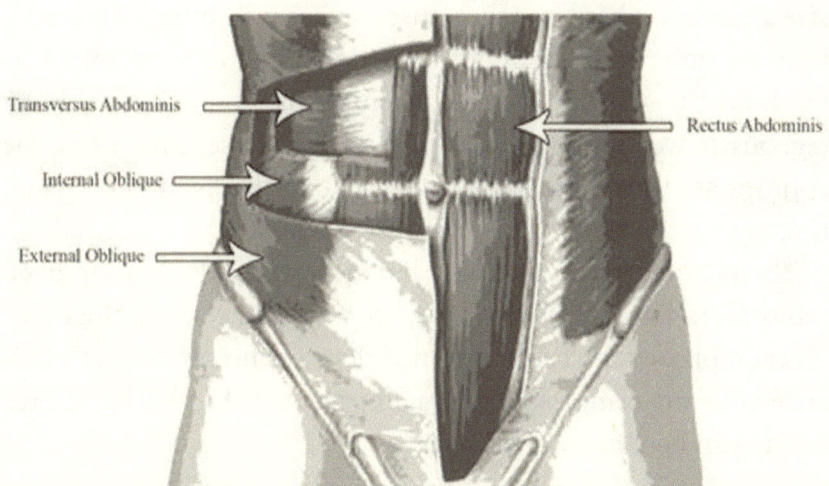

Back to core training...

We admit that strengthening the core muscles is a good idea; however, a weak core is often a symptom of a deeper and more serious problem.

The true problem occurs when the deep back muscles are not contracting together with the transverse abdominal muscles to stabilize your torso *(Hodges et al. 2003, 2594–2601; Cholewicki and VanVliett 2002, 99–105; Urquhart and Hodges 2005, 393–400).*

Here is an easy self check. While sitting or standing, place one hand on your belly and the other on your back. Now try to brace yourself as though someone is going to punch you in the gut.

Did you notice any movement in your low back? Now try again. Did you notice your back and belly moving at the same time?

In order to have a stable core that will allow your limbs to easily move throughout space, the timing of muscle activation in the front and back must be synchronized. When one of these muscles groups is not activated at the appropriate time, the body will quickly compensate by activating the more energy-expensive muscles. These are the muscles that will most commonly become tight or spasm due to being forced to work twice as hard. So the concept of strengthening the core is only advantageous if we train the body to activate those muscles at the appropriate time. And the only way to do that is to first ensure that your brain-body connection is balanced.

Being Neuromechanically Balanced will allow your deep multifidi to know when and how to properly activate. Once this is accomplished by seeing a trained doctor who can properly balance your neuromechanical system, you will be able to receive maximum benefit from core training.

Dr. Stuart McGill, an internationally respected expert in spinal biomechanics, developed the following "Big Three" exercises.

1. Modified Curl-Up

Lay on your back with one knee bent and one knee straight—placing your pelvis in a neutral position while the core muscles are in optimal alignment. Place your hands under the arch of your back, and ensure that this arch is maintained throughout the curl-up. Start by bracing your abdomen—imagining that you're pulling your umbilicus (belly button) toward your spine—and ensure that you are able to breathe in and out while holding this brace.

If you cannot perform this part, then stop and practice this portion until you can successfully breathe while maintaining this position.

Once you have mastered abdominal bracing, then add the following...

Imagine that your spine, neck, and upper back are cemented and cannot move independently. Hold a fixed gaze on the ceiling, and lift your shoulder blades about thirty degrees off the floor and slowly return to the start position. While doing this, ensure that your chin is not poking too far forward by forcing your chin back. This will help engage those often neglected deep cervical neck flexors.

Perform three sets of ten to twelve repetitions.

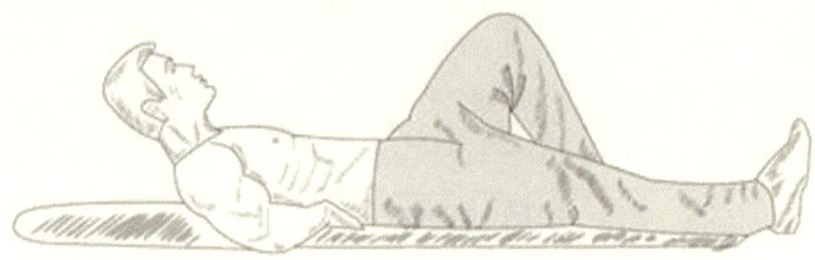

2. Side Bridge

Lie on your side, bend your knees to about 90 degrees and prop yourself up on your elbow. Ensure that your elbow is directly under your shoulder to avoid unwanted strain on the shoulder. Place your top hand on your bottom shoulder and keep your entire body aligned, trying not to rotate or to poke your pelvis forward or backward. Now brace your abdomen and squeeze your gluteals (buttock muscles) while lifting your hips off the ground. Make sure you are breathing, as this is not a breath-holding contest.

Hold this for position for eight to ten seconds, and repeat three times on the left side and three times on the right side.

If this becomes too easy, you can increase the intensity by placing the top hand on your top hip or in the air. But you must be sure your body is straight or else you'll defeat the purpose of the exercise.

You can also lie on your side and use your outstretched hand to support your body weight instead of your elbow. As always, be sure that your hand is properly aligned with your shoulder and that your entire body is aligned. Change the placement of your hand as your level of ability safely allows. This would progress from on the opposite shoulder to on the same side hip then reaching toward the ceiling with fingertips straight and palms forward.

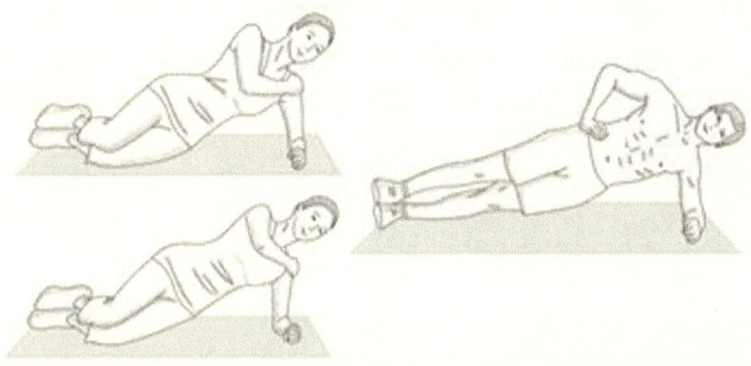

3. BIRD DOG

Start on your hands and knees. Place your hands shoulder-width apart and your knees hip-width apart. Make sure that your hands are directly underneath your shoulders and that your knees are directly under your hips. Maintain a neutral, aligned spine by preventing your back from dipping downward or arching upward. Then brace through your abdomen (belly button to spine), and squeeze with your gluteals while ensuring you are able to breathe in and out easily.

Once you have tightened your abdominal and buttocks muscles, lift your right arm in front of you until it is level with your shoulder. At the same time, extend your left leg straight back until it is level with your hips, squeezing your gluteals, and keeping your hips square with the floor. Return to the starting position in a slow and controlled manner, then perform the same action but with the opposite arm and leg. This counts as one repetition.

Perform three sets of eight to ten repetitions.

For an additional challenge, instead of putting your hands and knees back down on the ground between repetitions, try simply sweeping the floor and performing the next repetition right away, or draw a square with your arm or leg while it is in the air, and then sweep the floor.

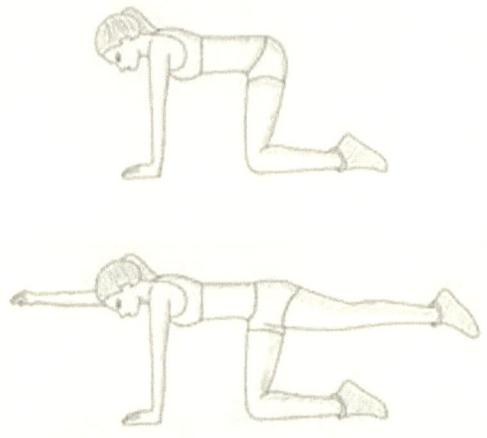

In Dr. McGill's book, Low Back Disorders: Evidence Based Prevention and Rehabilitation 2nd edition, he stated the preceding three exercises are "just a small selection of safe spine core exercises, yet are essential to master and perform in order to maintain great spinal stability."*(McGill 2002)*.

These exercises can also be used as a warm-up to your regular exercise routine. There are always ways to make each exercise harder as your stability and mobility improve. Just be patient, and remember "spinal stability before distal mobility." This translates to not being able to efficiently move your arms, hands, feet or legs (which are away from (or distal to) your spine) unless you first have a stabilized spine. It would otherwise be similar to driving a car with the tires out of alignment.

CHAPTER 22

MAKING YOUR WORLD
A SAFER PLACE

HOW TO DECREASE THE IMPACT OF
ENVIRONMENTAL STRESSORS

U p until now we have talked about the options that you and a trained doctor have to improve your Neuromechanical Imbalances and decrease the significant chronic stressors that contribute to the chronic stress cycle.

But what about all those environmental stressors that are out of our direct control?

The following are suggestions that we give to our patients to further reduce the chronic stressors in life. Take a look at some of the ways we have found to be effective to reduce the stressors in our air, water, lights, mental thoughts, and electromagnetic fields around our homes.

If you recall, acute stressors are vital for our survival in a stressful environment; otherwise, we would not survive the acute stressors. However, we are not designed to be under chronic stress. Nor were we designed to deal with acute fight-or-flight situations day in and day out, for weeks to months or even years. Unfortunately, this has become a recurring theme in many people's lives, which is why so many chronic conditions have developed.

Since we have this information, it is important to regulate stressors as much as possible. And the best way to begin this process is in your own home.

AIR WE BREATHE

Now of course the quality of air we breathe is an external factor that is not usually in our own control, unless you find avoiding places with more pollutants in the air an option. Realistically, though, that is not always an option.

On the other hand, you can make the choice to change the air quality in your home by purchasing an air purifier. Now maybe you are not home all day because you're like the majority of people who are either at work or out enjoying retirement, but what about when you sleep? Having an air purifier in your room (and children's rooms) will allow at least eight to nine hours (hopefully) of breathing in fresh, clean air per night.

We don't have any one brand of air purifier that we like best, but we would recommend ones that have a HEPA (high efficiency particulate air) filter. These ensure that the air is being properly filtrated.

Your other option could be to walk around with a personal air purifier around your neck at all times. We're kidding, of course. For the rest of us who do not find that to be a reasonable option, a simple air purifier in the household would make a great change in the air quality we breathe.

WATER WE DRINK

An adequate amount of clean water is critical to your health and fairly easy to obtain. There are only two questions to consider when it comes to your water consumption.

- What kind of water should you drink (tap, well, filtered, spring, mineral)?
- How much water should you drink?

The answers are fairly straightforward. Drinking either filtered tap water or filtered spring or mineral water is important to avoid harmful contaminants. Even mountain spring water can contain harmful contaminants if it's not filtered.

The safest and cheapest solution for most people is to filter their own tap water. You can filter your water with a pitcher filter (like a Brita® or Pur® brand), or you can install a water filter under your kitchen sink or on your water main.

The key to filtration is making sure you have an activated carbon filter (also known as a charcoal filter). This type of filter pulls out the really nasty stuff like chlorine and other harmful toxins. Paper filters alone just don't get the job done. Most good filters have a paper filter and an activated carbon filter.

A reverse osmosis filtration system is a more effective, albeit more expensive, water system. For those with extremely bad tap water, this would be the best option.

How much water you drink depends on your weight and activity level, but should usually be somewhere between six to ten cups a day. Other beverages that have water in them (soda, coffee, tea, and juice) do not count. Make sure you are drinking at least six cups of water every day whether or not you feel thirsty. As we age our thirst response decreases. You may not get thirsty, but you still need water.

In fact most of us have trained our bodies to believe we are hungry when we are actually thirsty. This is because we have trained our brains to think that we must eat in order to get the water that we need. While eating good healthy foods (as mentioned in the energy-restoration diet section) will supply fluid, it isn't a bad idea to actually take a drink of water to see if that decreases your hunger. Our bodies are composed of 60 percent water, so drinking more filtered water instead of sugary, carbonated beverages is always a better idea. And dehydration is a common chronic stressor to our bodies.

LIGHT WE SEE

More often than not, we are using Thomas Edison's (and others) invention of the light bulb once there is no longer daylight. You have already learned about the importance of getting sunlight to regulate circadian rhythms in the deep sleep chapter. Sunlight also has beneficial effects within the cells of our bodies. Sunlight provides important signaling to the hypothalamus (the brain's brain) about regulating automatic and metabolic processes. We could never enjoy the late-night rides, nightlife activities, or various other enjoyments that occur once the sun goes down if it were not for artificial lighting. Most importantly, we would not be able to see to maneuver around a building while at work or in a section of the house that is devoid of nearby windows.

That's why it is important to resort to the next best option... full spectrum lighting.

Full spectrum lights (although more expensive) display the entire wavelength of light, from infrared to near-ultraviolet. This type of lighting seeks to duplicate the light from the sun, which is considered full spectrum. These indoor lights dependably give off the full spectrum of light, regardless of the weather, time of day, or atmospheric conditions.

So if you are unable to receive adequate sunlight (which unfortunately many do not), this is the go-to option.

DEVELOPING AN ATTITUDE OF APPRECIATION

As you have already learned, an overactive, chronic stress response is remarkably prevalent and detrimental in today's society. We have already discussed how to become more para-sympathetically driven through the DICE protocol, and we have explored how to become neuromechanically balanced. Now we have yet another suggestion...gratitude.

When you are consciously focusing on what you are grateful for, you simply eliminate the opportunity to focus on things that are stressful.

Have you ever heard of "placing things out in the universe" or "leaving it in God's hands"? And when you have least expected it, that thing that was creating stress or anxiety in your life resolved. Well, expressing gratitude is a great alternative to focusing on life's stressors.

Start creating a habit of writing 10-20 things that you are thankful for. You can also choose to mentally list them, share them with a significant other, or say them as a prayer. The choice doesn't matter as much as the creating the attitude of thankful-ness and joy that you seek to develop. You can easily put this into practice first thing in the morning or directly before going to bed.

The act of performing this process will bring a smile to your face. The more consistent you are with this routine, the more your brain will go on autopilot and provide positive thoughts. This habit will work to not only quiet your sympathetics (fight or flight) when they are not needed but will actually start to make you feel good and seem more charismatic to others. It's a win-win outcome!

The next time you lay your head down to rest, try counting your blessings rather than counting sheep.

PEMF THERAPY—WE LIVE IN AN ELECTROMAGNETIC WORLD

With our technologically driven world, it is no wonder so many people have become entirely consumed in social media on their computers, tablets, or smart phones. Our society is sitting more, which is contributing to the development of chronic diseases and autoimmunities, having poor posture, and being more depressed. And our bodies have also been flooded with heavy amounts of electromagnetic waves. These electromagnetic waves are everywhere due to our amazing, yet overwhelmingly populated, world of electronic devices.

In fact, until recently, we were not allowed to use cell phones while on the airplane due to the worry that airliners' calls would interfere with ground-based communications. We're not suggesting that our bodies are breaking down due to our need for technology, but we certainly don't think it helps our already wound-up stress responses. Our bodies are a form of electrically charged machines that can benefit from healing from intermittent electric fields. This is why we suggest the use of Quantron Resonance System's Pulsed Electro Magnetic Field Therapy (PEMF) for home use.

There has been strong evidence supporting the use of PEMF therapy for chronic low back pain and sciatica. We have found it to be a valuable home therapy for our patients with severe spinal decay.

Doctors in Europe have used PEMF for a number of conditions since the 1970s. It is extremely safe, pain free, and has an extremely small chance of causing negative side effects (so small that many experts consider it to be free of side effects). PEMF has actually been used to treat neurological disorders since the 1990s. It has been clinically shown to speed the recovery of damaged nerves *(Ito and Bassett 1983, 283–90; Orgel and O'Brien and Murray 1984, 173–83; Raji 1984, 105–12).*

In addition to speeding up recovery time for damaged nerves, PEMF has also been shown in clinical studies to reduce pain associated with peripheral neuropathy and other chronic diseases *(Musaev and Guseinova and Imanverdieva 2003, 745–52).* In fact a study using PEMF on patients with diabetic neuropathy showed that treatment every day for only twelve minutes caused a reduction in pain, an increase in vibration sensation, and an increase in muscular strength in 85 percent of patients *(Pawluk 2003).*

Despite the great results seen in studies, PEMF is not yet a common treatment in the United States—mostly due to US doctors' lack of understanding about the different modalities of PEMF therapy. If you're interested in learning about how this device works and what unit to choose, refer to Appendix C.

CLOSING LETTER BY THE AUTHORS: THE KEYS TO VIGOROUS HEALTH

We hope by now you are as excited as we are to know that you do not have to live with pain for the rest of your life and that you do not have take drugs to reduce pain. We're not suggesting that there is a cure-all for any chronic disease pattern or pain symptoms, but most (if not all) have stemmed from the body becoming incapable of being able to appropriately heal and react to our modern world.

We have described various aspects of your environment and how they can negatively impact your health. We have also offered suggestions on how to manage and decrease these chronic stressors and have shared an effective strategy for treating the underlying cause of your low back pain.

Your first step is to find a doctor who understands these principles and will work with you on balancing your nervous system as well as helping you to reduce the chronic stressors in your life. From there you can use the DICE protocol included in part three of this book to take matters into your own hands. This will not eliminate your Neuromechanical Imbalances, but it will decrease your chronic stress load.

There are many lifestyle changes included in our DICE protocol that may seem overwhelming at first, but you can take them in small bites. You can gain tremendous benefits without having to do everything. Lowering your stress load by starting with just a few strategies will have a cumulative effect. You'll be surprised at how a few changes in your lifestyle can have a noticeable impact.

Don't let your chronic low back pain put the brakes on your life. No matter your age or how severe your condition, there is always room for improvement. Our wish is that you will be proactive in your search for answers to your condition. We hope that this book has given you some of those answers as well as strategies that you can use to improve the quality of your life.

An old proverb says, "The best time to plant a tree is twenty years ago. The second-best time is now."

Now is the best time to begin lowering your chronic stress, balancing your spine, and moving toward vigorous health.

Yours in health and vitality,
Drs. Russ, Lee, and Natalie

RECOMMENDED READING

Why Zebras Don't Get Ulcers (St. Martin's Press) by Robert M. Sapolsky. This book is a great resource if you want to learn more about how the *stress response* leads to degeneration and disease. However the author focuses mostly on psychological stressors, for a better look at physical stressors I recommend the book below.

Rewire Your Brain by John b. Arden, Ph.D. With the author's knowledge of the brain actually being "soft-wired" rather than "hard-wired", he is able to provide ways of developing mental connections that promote good habits while shutting off those that support bad habits. It can help quite the brain to minimize anxiety, conquer fear, and enhance the brain's longevity in order to "live a vibrant life."

The Chronic Stress Crisis: How Stress Is Destroying Your Health & What You Can Do To Stop It (AuthorHouse) by William G. Timmins, N.D. In this book you'll get a better understanding of the various physical environmental stressors which can lead to the *continuous stress response*.

Grain Brain by Dr. David Perlmutter thoroughly addresses the damage that gluten and carbs are doing to our brains. He outlines and provides research on how our society's skewed view on the need for carbs can be leading to various chronic diseases and symptoms including, depression, dementia, headaches, ADHD, anxiety and more.

Wheat Belly: Lose the Wheat, Lose the Weight, and Find Your Path Back to Health (Rodale) by William Davis, MD. This book is a great explanation of why wheat and related grains should be avoided even if you aren't gluten reactive. It goes into the detail of how wheat has changed of the past 100 years and the effect those changes are having on human health.

Perfect Breathing: Transform Your Life One Breath at a Time (Sterling) by Al Lee and Don Campbell. From this book you'll learn more details on how proper breathing can boost the amount of oxygen in your blood, improve circulation, and reduce stress. It also contains several breathing exercises you can use in addition to the ones given in chapter 19.

Stand Taller Live Longer by Dr. Stephen G. Weiniger provides insight on how posture affects your life now, 20 and even 30 years from now. He illustrates and discusses a 7-week program will strengthen your posture to keep you" moving well and pain-free" by doing his provided posture exercises just 10 minutes a day.

The Blue Zones by Dan Buettner is a great book on a researcher who hunted around the world for extremely healthy populations He researched several different areas of the world that had the highest percentage of people over one hundred years of age and came to some fascinating conclusions health throughout the ages.

ADDITIONAL RESOURCES

Platelet Rich Plasma (PRP) Therapy for those that are interested in this form of therapy, we recommend Dwight James, M.D. from Porterville, CA (559)781-3014.

Sciatica Exercises & Home Treatment: Simple, Effective Care For Sciatica and Piriformis Syndrome by George Best, DC. As the title states, this is a great adjunct for at-home strategies of controlling sciatic pain.

Mind Body Tool Kit by Andrew Weil, MD is an insightful source of learning how to heal from the inside out. In this tool-kit, Dr Weil provides an audio guide of sound and music in addition to a colorful instructional booklet that opens the path to self-healing in the convenience of your own home.

www.Allrecipes.com: this is a terrific website to find recipes for your ATP Diet, simply go to the search window enter the dish or food you would like to prepare (such as cupcake) and click on "ingredient" and list the ingredients you want to exclude (such as milk and grains) and it will give you a list of recipes!

www.LabTestOnline.org : this is a "Patient Centered" website that describes various lab tests, what they are used for, and what they mean. The information on this site is based on "lab values" and does not differentiate between lab and functional values.

<u>www.cyrexlabs.com</u> : We use this lab for some of my testing, there's a short 3 minute video on its website titled, "Gut-Brain Connection", that does a very good job of describing the problem of Leaky Gut and how its related to systemic inflammation (silent inflammation) and disease.

<u>www.ThePaleoDiet.com</u>: This site has resources for the Paleo-Diet which is very similar to the ATP Diet which we recommend you follow. On this site you'll find many recipe ideas, as well as research on how diet affects silent inflammation.

DOCTOR RESOURCES

Low Back Disorders: Evidence Based Prevention and Rehabilitation 2nd edition by Stuart McGill, PhD. His textbook is designed to educate the reader about the basis of the lumbar spine and how it functions to provide stability throughout the rest of the body. He continues by providing the research and most importantly, dozens of colorful pages that full of exercises that are designed to regain stability, improve function and performance no matter the level of experience.

Low Back Syndromes- Integrated Clinical Management by Craig E. Morris, DC, DACRB, FAFIC, CSCS. He collaborated with multiple professionals of varying disciplines to determine the available clinical options for low back conditions. The disciplines range from chiropractic to osteopathy and physical therapy to medicine (and more.) It is a practical guide of the standards of practice all in one source.

Functional Neurology for the Manual Practitioner by Randy Beck, DC, PhD, DACNB, FAAFN, FACFN. This book is your functional neurology resource. It provides darn near everything you need and more for having a thorough understanding of neurology and how you can look at its inner workings from the outside. What's more, is that it also provides some insightful approaches to patient management and treatment for those that you encounter in your office.

Rehabilitation of the Spine: A Practitioners Manual by Craig Liebenson, DC. This particular book offers step by step guidelines for the managing and rehabilitation of spinal conditions also with a multi-disciplinary approach. More importantly, this book evidence and how to apply it to everyday practice.

Why Isn't My Brain Working? A Revolutionary Understanding of Brain Decline and Effective Strategies to Recover Your Brain's Health by Datis Kharrazian, DHSc., DC, MS. He runs through the neurology of and physiology of why the brain can decline regardless of age. He provides insightful sources and guidance on how simple diet and lifestyle changes and nutritional therapy can profoundly impact your brain health and thus the quality of your life.

The Innate Diet & Natural Hygiene by James L Chestnut, M.Sc, D.C, C.C.W.P. This book is within a series of his Wellness Practice collection of eating, moving, and thinking well. Dr Chestnut provides an eye-opening perspective on health and the keys to achieving wellness through our dietary intake. Though it is written to be aided with chiropractic care, he provides neurophysiological evidence for why our current diet is hurting us and answers to how we can return back to our roots of eating well.

Neurobehavioral Disorders of Childhood: An Evolutionary Perspective by Drs. Robert Melillo and Gerry Leisman. This book provides an evolutionary basis on the human neurology. It is densely packed with research and information that explains the inner workings of the brain and how hemispheric dominance or disconnections can alter childhood development. The authors emphasize how hemispheric treatment is the key to correcting these developmental disorders found in children.

Apex Seminars - (800-736-4381)—Apex sponsored seminars are open to all health care professionals (MD's, DO's, DC's, Nurses, etc.) and cover topics such as functional blood chemistry, functional endocrinology, and nutritional courses. The seminar materials are well referenced, in depth, and practical. This would be a good "first step" for any doctor that wants to start integrating a more functional approach into their practice.

Carrick Institute - (321-868-6464) carrickinstitute.org— The Carrick Institute offers a program of study in Clinical Neurology. Like Apex Seminars, it is also open to DC's, MD's, DO's, etc. The program takes approximately two years to complete, although additional courses are added yearly throughout the country (and world). The focus of the program is on Functional Neurology and its various applications that can be applied in you practice the next week..

Quantron Resonance System (QRS)—Pulsed Electro Magenetic Field Therapy qrs.com QRS is the gold standard in PEMF therapy. Their units are the most researched and proven PEMF units on the market today. If you are looking to incorporate PEMF therapy in your practice I suggest looking into QRS's units first.

APPENDIX A

ENERGY-RESTORATION DIET

ENERGY-RESTORATION DIET FRIENDLY FOODS

It can often be difficult to avoid dwelling on the foods you can't have when you're on a diet. For that reason we've included this list of ordinary foods that you can have. Hopefully this list will help in meal planning and will encourage you to follow the diet.

Starches
- Butternut squash
- Sweet potatoes
- Yams

Vegetables
- All cooking greens, including collard greens, mustard greens, kale, chard, etc.
- All salad greens, including all types of lettuce, spinach, arugula, etc.
- All squashes, including zucchini, yellow squash, acorn, butternut, pumpkin, etc.
- Asparagus
- Beets
- Broccoli

- Brussels sprouts
- Cabbage (bok choy, red, napa, regular, etc.)
- Carrots
- Celery
- Garlic
- Onions
- Parsnips
- Radishes
- Turnips

Fruits
- Apples
- Apricots
- Avocado
- Bananas
- Blackberries
- Blueberries
- Cherries
- Coconut
- Cranberries
- Dates
- Grapefruits
- Grapes
- Kiwi
- Mango
- Nectarines
- Olives
- Oranges
- Peaches
- Pears
- Pineapples
- Plums

- Pomegranates
- Raspberries
- Strawberries

Nuts—Peanuts are *not* allowed during phase one.
- Almonds
- Brazil nuts
- Cashews
- Chestnuts
- Hazelnuts
- Pecans
- Pine nuts
- Pistachios
- Macadamias
- Walnuts

All Meats—Preferably buy unprocessed meats; however, if you choose to eat processed meats, like sausages or canned meats, be sure to check labels for gluten, MSG, or sugar. This does not include breaded meats.
- All poultry—chicken, turkey, duck, etc.
- All seafood
- Beef
- Bison
- Pork
- Venison

Fermented Foods
- Kimchi
- Olives
- Pickle relish, pickled asparagus, onions, peppers, etc.
- Pickles

- Sauerkraut

Condiments
- Canola oil
- Coconut oil
- Mustards that don't have sugar added
- Olive oil
- Safflower oil
- Vinegars—white and red wine vinegar, balsamic vinegar, apple cider vinegar, etc.

Seasonings—Most individual seasonings are fine, except chili powder, paprika, and true peppers like crushed red pepper (not the pepper in your pepper shaker). Those particular spices are not allowed because they include vegetables from the nightshade family and can be slightly inflammatory in nature. Beware of seasoning packets or premade seasonings, which include many spices but don't list all ingredients. These packets often contain MSG (to falsely lower their sodium content) or wheat (to thicken sauces).
- Allspice
- Basil
- Caraway
- Cilantro
- Cinnamon
- Clove
- Coriander
- Cumin
- Dill
- Fennel
- Garlic powder

- Marjoram
- Nutmeg
- Onion powder
- Oregano
- Parsley
- Pepper
- Rosemary
- Salt
- Thyme
- Turmeric
- And any other spice you want

APPENDIX B

GLYCEMIC INDEX AND LOAD FOR THE ENERGY-RESTORATION DIET

All foods have a unique impact on blood glucose levels when eaten. Some foods cause a large and quick rise in blood glucose and others have a very modest effect on blood glucose. As you know from reading chapter twenty-two, keeping your blood glucose level low and stable is very important if you want to decrease your chronic stress load.

Keeping your blood glucose level low and stable helps lower inflammation and boost energy levels. Keep in mind, when we say keep your blood glucose low, we are referring to a safe, low level for you. If you are diabetic, your low may be much higher than a young, healthy individual. The goal is to keep your blood glucose low and steady relative to what is the normal range for you. With that in mind, it is important for you to work with your health-care provider to define what level is good for you.

Paying attention to the impact each food in a given meal has on your blood glucose level is the best way to manage your blood sugar. It is also an important part of making the energy-restoration diet work for you. Using the glycemic index and glycemic load of foods is a good starting point to track the impact meals have on your blood glucose and to build smarter meals.

The glycemic index of a food is determined by giving human test subjects a given amount of a food then testing their blood glucose levels as the carbohydrates in the food are digested and absorbed into the blood stream. Each food is given a score based on how quickly it raises blood sugar, relative to eating pure glucose. The value given for each food is measured on a scale of zero to one hundred. One hundred is the value given to pure glucose. All other foods are lower.

Using the glycemic index of foods is problematic in certain cases, because it is determined by giving subjects rather large servings of foods that are ordinarily eaten in small quantities. This problem arises because the test is based on a test subject eating whatever quantity of a given food is needed to have a total of fifty grams of available carbohydrates (indigestible fiber doesn't count).

For example, test subjects would only need to eat one large baked potato to get fifty grams of carbohydrates, while they would have to eat roughly one and one-half pounds of carrots to get fifty grams of carbohydrates. For this reason carrots are misleadingly high on the glycemic index. Carrots aren't really carbohydrate dense, but the carbohydrates they do contain are quickly absorbed. Even so, few people could eat a quantity of carrots large enough to cause their blood glucose to skyrocket.

This nuance to the calculation of glycemic index can be very misleading to the public. Tables of glycemic index values of common foods are available in many places, and misleading results like the issue with carrots has led to much confusion.

Glycemic load was created to fix this problem. The glycemic load is an attempt to determine how a particular serving size of a food will affect blood glucose. Because it is serving-size dependent it is much more useful in meal planning. Glycemic load values are still based on the glycemic index research, but by adding in serving size values, they become much more useful for the general public.

The website www.mendosa.com/gilists.htm includes a large list of foods and where they fall within the glycemic load and index chart.

For meal-building purposes, you want to eat large quantities of vegetables that have low-glycemic load values. If you eat vegetables or fruits that have medium-glycemic load values, you should eat smaller portions. (Your plate should have some empty space on it.) When eating high-glycemic fruits and vegetables along with your lean protein, you should have a lot of empty space on your plate.

APPENDIX C

PULSED ELECTROMAGNETIC FIELD THERAPY (PEMF)

HOW IT WORKS

Quantron Resonance System's PEMF units work both directly and indirectly to relieve pain and promote the healing of cells within the body. First, PEMF therapy increases the threshold of pain sensitivity in treated areas. Second, it improves the movement of calcium ions (necessary for neuron firing), enabling cells, especially neurons, to more easily regain their proper membrane potentials.

This therapy has a number of indirect effects on healing, including increasing the movement of ions inside of cells, as well as increasing the movement of ions into and out of cells, and improving the intake of nutrients and the removal of waste on a cellular level. The PEMF therapy also improves blood circulation and cellular oxygenation and has been shown to positively affect autonomic balance after exercise *(Grote et al. 2007, 495–502)*.

Because PEMF improves circulation, it is great for reducing inflammation. Lastly, because it aids in the movement of ions, PEMF improves a cell's ability to produce ATP (the cellular source of energy). In fact, QRS's PEMF units have an international patent for their ability to transport ions across cell membranes, something no other PEMF manufacturer has been able to do.

What's more, most of the benefits of PEMF therapy have global effects on the body. In other words, this therapy doesn't just target your pain. This is a huge benefit. This ability to work deeply within your body's tissues makes PEMF therapy an indispensable tool for those suffering from many chronic diseases. That is why this device can be of significant value to many of those who suffer from low back pain.

CHOOSING A PEMF UNIT

Keep in mind that not all PEMF devices are created equal. There is a high degree of variability in the effectiveness of these devices depending upon the manufacturer. From our own research and clinical experience, we have found PEMF units made by Quantron Resonance Systems (QRS) to be the best option. A large amount of the research done on the effectiveness of PEMF in treating a multitude of conditions has been done using QRS devices.

In fact, QRS's PEMF units have over two hundred research papers supporting their effectiveness for a wide variety of health problems, making them the most researched units on the market today. Quantron Resonance Systems also holds three international patents on proprietary technology. QRS was also chosen by the MIR Space Station to protect the Astronauts' decrease in bone density post space travel. Either way, we recommend choosing a device with a clear track record of success.

SELECTED REFERENCES

Adams, Case. 2011. *Breathing to Heal: The Science of Healthy Respiration.* Wilmington: Logical Books.

Alaedini A, et al. 2007. "Immune cross-reactivity in celiac disease: anti-gliadin antibodies bind to neuronal synapsin I." *Journal of Immunology* 178 (May): 6590–5.

Aleshukina AV. 2012. "Pathogenesis of intestinal dysbacteriosis." *Zh Mikrobiol Epidemiol Immunobiol* 3 (May–June): 74–8.

Alyas F, Turner M, Connell D. 2007. "MRI findings in the lumbar spines of asymptomatic, adolescent, elite tennis players." *BR J Sports Medicine* 41 (November): 836–41.

American Association of Neurological Surgeons. 2011. "Low Back Pain." (December) accessed at www.aans.org

Anders HJ, Andersen K, Stecher B. 2013. "The intestinal microbiota, a leaky gut, and abnormal immunity in kidney disease." *Kidney Int* (January) doi: 10.1038/ki.2012.440.

Argoff CE, Wheeler AH, Backonja MM, ed. 1998. "Spinal and radicular pain syndromes." *Philadelphia, WB Saunders: Neurologic Clinics* 833–45.

Binder DS, Nampiaparampil DE. 2009. "The provocative lumbar facet joint." *Current Review Musculoskeletal Medicine* 2 (March): 15–24.

Bob P. 2008. "Lateralized brain and neuroendocrine dysregulation as response to traumatic stress." *Neuro Endocrinol Lett* 29 (April): 185–91.

Borkan J, Van Tulder M, et al. 2002. "Advances in the field of low back pain in primary care. A report from the fourth International forum." *Spine* 27 (5): E128–132.

Bosma-den Boer MM, van Wetten ML, Pruimboom L. 2012. "Chronic inflammatory diseases are stimulated by current lifestyle: how diet, stress levels and medication prevent our body from recovering." *Nutrition & Metabolism* 9 (April): 32.

Brandenberger G, Weibel L. 2004. "The 24-h growth hormone rhythm in men: sleep and circadian influences questioned." *Journal of Sleep Research* 13 (September): 251–5.

Braun C. 2007. "Evolution of hemispheric specialization of antagonistic systems of management of the body's energy resources." *Laterality* 12(5): 397-427.

Brown, Kirsty, et al. 2012. "Diet Induced Dysbiosis of the Intestinal Microbiota and the Effects on Immunity and Disease." *Nutrients* 4 (August): 1095–1119.

Bures J, et al. 2010. "Small intestinal bacterial overgrowth syndrome." *World Journal of Gastroenterology* 16 (June): 2978–90.

Cailliet, Rene. 1987. *The Rejuvenation Strategy*. New York: Doubleday & Company.

Carney, Dana R. et al. 2010. "Power Posing: Brief Nonverbal Displays Affect Neuroendocrine Levels and Risk Tolerance." *Psychological Science* 21 (October): 1363–8.

Chestnut, James L. 2005. *The Innate State of Mind & Emotional Hygiene.* Victoria, British Columbia: Global Self Health Corp.

Chiappa GR, et al. 2008. "Inspiratory muscle training improves blood flow to resting and exercising limbs in patients with chronic heart failure." *Journal of the American College Cardiology* 51 (April): 1663–71.

Cholewicki J, VanVliet IJ. 2002. "Relative contribution of trunk muscles to the stability of the lumbar spine during isometric exertions." *Clin Biomech* 17(February): 99–105.

Cohen, S, et al. 2012. "Chronic stress, glucocorticoid receptor resistance, inflammation, and disease risk." *Proceedings of the National Academy of Science USA* 109 (April): 5995–9.

Courtney R, Cohen M, van Dixhoorn J. 2011. "Relationship between dysfunctional breathing patterns and ability to achieve target heart rate variability with features of 'coherence' during biofeedback." *Alternative Therapies in Health and Medicine* 17 (May–June): 38–44.

Crimmins and Beltrán-Sánchez. 2010. "Mortality and Morbidity Trends: Is There Compression of Morbidity?" *Journal of Gerontology.*

Diya RA. 1996. "Drug therapy for back pain. Which drugs help which patients?" *Spine* (December): 2840–9; discussion 2849–50.

Deyo RA. 1997. "Nonoperative treatment of low back disorders: differentiated useful from useless therapy." In *The Adult Spine: Principles and*

Practice, edited by JW Frymoyer, TB Ducker, NM Hadler, et al., 1777–93. Philadelphia: Lippincott-Raven.

Doidge, N. (2007) The brain that changes itself: stories of personal triumph from the frontiers of brain science, Penguin Books

Drago S, et al. 2006. "Gliadin, zonulin and gut permeability: Effects on celiac and non-celiac intestinal mucosa and intestinal cell lines." *Scandinavian Journal of Gastroenterology* 41 (April): 408–19.

DuPont AW, DuPont HL. 2011. "The intestinal microbiota and chronic disorders of the gut." *Nature Reviews. Gastroenterology & Hepatology* 8 (August): 523–31.

Eisenmann A, Murr C, Fuchs D, Ledochowski M. 2009. "Gliadin IgG antibodies and circulating immune complexes." *Scandinavian Journal of Gastroenterology* 44, (2): 168–71.

El Boustani S, et al. 1989. "Direct in vivo characterization of delta 5 desaturase activity in humans by deuterium labeling: effect of insulin." *Metabolism* 38 (April): 315–21.

Eskay-Auerbach, M. 2005. *Medical-legal aspects of the spine.* Tuscan, AZ: Lawyers and Judges Publishing Co.

Ferrari E, Cravello L, Muzzoni B, et al. 2001. "Age-related changes of the hypothalamic-pituitary-adrenal axis: pathophysiological correlates." *European Journal of Endocrinology* 144 (April): 319–29.

Fortuniak J, Jaskólski D, Tybor K, Komuński P, Zawirski M. 2005. "Role of proteoglycans and glycosaminoglycans in the intervertebral disc degeneration." *Neurol Neurochir Pol* 39 (July–August): 324–7.

Frymoyer JW. 1988. "Back pain and sciatica." *New England Journal of Medicine* 318 (February 14): 291–300.

Gibbons S. 2014. "Neurocognitive and Sensory Motor Deficits represent and important sub classification for musculoskeletal disorders-central nervous system coordination."*BMC Musculoskeletal Disorders* 15:52.

Glei DA, Goldman N, Chuang YL, Weinstein M. 2007. "Do chronic stressors lead to physiological dysregulation? Testing the theory of allostatic load." *Psychosomatic Medicine* 69 (November): 769–76.

Golman, N. 2007. "Allostatic load: measurement issues and future directions." *Institute of Behavioral Sciences.* Summer Course in Biodemography (June)

Gonzalez-Burgos I, Perez-Vega MI, Beas-Zarate C, 2001. "Neonatal exposure to monosodium glutamate induces cell death and dendritic hypotrophy in rat prefrontocortical pyramidal neurons." *Neuroscience Letters* 297 (January): 69–72.

Ludvigsson JF, Olsson T, Ekbom A, Montgomery SM. 2007. "A population-based study of coeliac disease, neurodegenerative and neuro-inflammatory diseases." *Alimentary Pharmacology & Therapeutics* 25 (June): 1317–27.

Gose EE, Naguszewski WK, Naguszewski RK. 1998. "Vertebral Axial Decompression Therapy for Pain associated with herniated or degenerated discs, degenerated discs, or facet syndrome: An outcome study." *Journal of Neurological Research* 20 (April): 186-190.

Grote V, et al. 2007. "Short-term effects of pulsed electromagnetic fields after physical exercise are dependent on autonomic tone before exposure." *European Journal of Applied Physiology* 101 (November): 495–502.

Gruber HE, Hoelscher GL, Ingram JA, Hanley EN. 2012. "Genome-wide analysis of pain-, nerve- and neurotrophin-related gene expression in the degenerating human annulus." *Mol Pain* 8 (September 10): 63.

Gruenewald TL et al. 2006. "Combinations of biomarkers predictive of later life mortality." *PNAS* 103: 14158-14163.

Hadjivassiliou M, et al. 2006. "Neuropathy associated with gluten sensitivity." *Journal of Neurology Neurosurgery & Psychiatry* 77 (November): 1262–6.

Hart RP, Wade J, Martelli MF. 2003. "Cognitive Impairment in Patients with chronic Pain: The significance of Stress."*Current Pain and Headache Reports.* 7:116-226.

Hodges P, Kaigle-Holm A, Holm S. et al. 2003. "Intervertebral stiffness of the spine is increased by evoked contraction of tranversus abdominis and the diaphragm: In vivo porcine studies." *Spine* 28: 2594–2601.

Hussain A, Erdek M. 2014. "Interventional Pain Management for Failed Back Surgery Syndrome." *Pain Practice* 14 (1): 64–78.

Institute of Medicine of the National Academies. *Physiologic, Psychologic, and Psychosocial Effects of Deployment-Related Stress Vol. 6. 2008.* Washington, DC: National Academies Press.

Ito H, Bassett CA. 1983. "Effect of weak, pulsing electromagnetic fields on neural regeneration in the rat." *Clinical Orthopaedics and Related Research* 181 (December): 283–90.

Itz CJ, et al. 2013. "Clinical course of nonspecific low back pain: A systematic review of prospective cohort studies set in primary care." *European Journal of Pain* 17: 5–15.

Jensen MC, Brant-Zawadzki MN, Obuchowski N, Modic MT, Malkasian D, Ross JS. 1994. "Magnetic resonance imaging of the lumbar spine in people without back pain." *New England Journal of Medicine* 331 (2): 69–73.

Kapreli E. 2009. "Respiratory dysfunction in chronic neck pain patients. A pilot study." *Cephalalgia* 29 (7): 701–10.

Karatsoreos IN, McEwen BS. 2011. "Pshychobiological allostasis: resistance, resilience and vulnerability." *Trends in Cognitive Sciences* 15 (December)12: 579-582.

Karlamangla AS et al. (2002). "Allostatic load as a predictor of functional decline: MacArthur studies of successful aging." *Journal of Clinical Epidemiology* 55(7): 696-710.

Krock E, Rosenzweig DH, Chabot-Doré AJ, Jarzem P, Weber MH, Ouellet JA, Stone LS, Haglund L. 2014. "Painful, degenerating intervertebral discs up-regulate neurite sprouting and CGRP through nociceptive factors." *J Cell Mol Med* (March 20):1213-25.

Kumar V, Abbas AK, Fausto N. 2005. *Robbins and Cotran: Pathologic Basis of Disease*. 7th ed. Philadelphia: Elsevier Saunders.

Lee, Al and Don Campbell. 2009. *Perfect Breathing*. New York: Sterling.

Lee MJ, et al. 2012. "Risk factors for medical complication after spine surgery: a multivariate analysis of 1,591 patients." *The Spine Journal* 12:197–206.

Leproult R, Copinschi G, Buxton O, Van Cauter E. 1997. "Sleep loss results in an elevation of cortisol levels the next evening." *Sleep* 20 (October): 865–70.

Ludke RL, Rothe K. August 2014. "Allostatic Load and its Utilization in Clinical Practice." accessed at www.allostatix.com.

Malanga G, Wolf E. 2008. "Evidence-informed management of chronic low back pain with non-steroidal anti-inflammatory drugs, muscle relaxants, and simple analgesics." *Spine J* 8 (January–February): 173–84.

Manev H, Favaron M, Guidotti A, Costa E. 1989. "Delayed increase of Ca2+ influx elicite." *Molecular Pharmacology* 36 (July): 106–12.

Matsumoto M, Okada E, Toyama Y, Fujiwara H, Momoshima S, Takahata T. 2013. "Tandem age–related lumbar and cervical intervertebral disc changes in asymptomatic subjects." *Eur Spine J* 4 (April): 708–13.

McEwen BS, Stellar E. 1993. "Stress and the individual. Mechanisms leading to disease." *Archives of Internal Medicine* 27 (September): 2093–101.

McEwen, BS. 1998. "Protective and damaging effects of stress mediators." *The New England Journal of Medicine.* 338(3), 171-180.

McEwen, BS. 2002. "Sex, stress and the hippocampus: allotstasis, allostatic load and the aging process." *Neurobiology of Aging.* 23, 921-939.

McEwen BS. 2006. "Sleep deprivation as a neurobiologic and physiologic stressor: Allostasis and allostatic load." *Metabolism* 55 (October): S20–3.

McEwen, BS, Wingfield, J. 2010. "What's in a name? Integrating homeostasis, allostasis and stress." *Hormones and Behavior.* 57(2):105.

McEwen BS, Gianaros PJ. 2011. "Stress- and allostasis-induced brain plasticity." *Annu Rev Med* 62: 431–45.

McKwen, B, Nasveld, P, Palmer, M, Anderson, R. 2012. *Allostatic Load: A Review of Literature.* Canberra: Department of Veterans' affairs.

Miyake K, Tanaka T, McNeil PL. 2007. "Lectin-based food poisoning: a new mechanism of protein toxicity." *PLoS One* 2 (August): e687.

Mooney V. 1987. "Where is the pain coming from? 1986 Presidential address of the International Society for the Study of the Lumbar Spine." *Spine* 12 (October): 754–9.

Moore, M et al. 2011. "Mind-body skills for regulating the autonomic nervous system." *Defense Centers of Excellence for Psychological Health and Traumatic Brain Injury* 2 (June): 1-20.

Musaev AV, Guseinova SG, Imanverdieva SS. 2003. "The use of pulsed electromagnetic fields with complex modulation in the treatment of patients with diabetic polyneuropathy." *Neuroscience & Behavioral Physiology* 33 (October): 745–52.

Nachbar MS, Oppenheim JD. 1980. "Lectins in the United States diet: a survey of lectins in commonly consumed foods and a review of the literature." *American Journal of Clinical Nutrition* 33 (November): 2338–45.

Novak, Janice. 2006. *Posture, Get It Straight.* Andover: Expert Publishing.

Orgel MG, O'Brien WJ, Murray HM. 1984. "Pulsing electromagnetic field therapy in nerve regeneration: an experimental study in the cat." *Plastic & Reconstructive Surgery* 73 (February): 173–83.

Pascual-Leone A, Amedi A, Fregni F, Merabet LB. 2005. "The plastic human brain cortex." *Annual Review of Neuroscience* 28: 377–401

Pascual-Leone A, et al. 2011. "Characterizing brain cortical plasticity and network dynamics across the age-span in health and disease with TMS-EEG and TMS-fMRI." *Brain Topography* 24 (October): 302–15.

Paul M, Garg K. 2012. "The effect of heart rate variability biofeedback on performance psychology of basketball players." *Applied Psychophysiology and Biofeedback* 37 (June): 131–44.

Pawluk, W. 2003. "Pain Management with Pulsed Electromagnetic Field (PEMF) Treatment." (March)

PEPPER User's Guide, Twelfth Edition: Twelfth edition: Short Term Acute Care Program for Evaluating Payment Patterns Electronic Report. 2013. TMF Health Quality Institute.

Quévrain E, Seksik P. 2013. "Intestinal microbiota: From antibiotic-associated diarrhea to inflammatory bowel diseases." *Presse Med* 42 (January): 45–51.

Rajeswaran G, Turner M, Gissane C, Healy JC. 2014. "MRI findings in the lumbar spines of asymptomatic elite junior tennis players." *Skeletal Radiol* 43 (July): 925–32.

Raji AM. 1984. "An experimental study of the effects of pulsed electromagnetic field (Diapulse) on nerve repair." *Journal of Hand Surgery* 9 (June): 105–12.

Sapolsky, Robert M. 1996. "Stress, Glucocorticoids, and Damage to the Nervous System: The Current State of Confusion." *Stress* 1 (July): 1–19.

Sapolsky, Robert M. 2004. *Why Zebras Don't Get Ulcers*. New York: St. Martin's.

Scully, Lynn C. 2010. *"Association Between Alostatic Load and Arthritis NHANES Adults."* Department of Epidemiology and Biostatistics.

Sears, Barry. 2005. *The Anti-Inflammation Zone: Reversing the Silent Epidemic That's Destroying Our Health*. New York: HarperCollins.

Seaward, Brian. 2011. *Managing Stress*. Burlington: Jones and Bartlett.

Seress L, Lazar G, Kosaras B, Robertson RT. 1984. "Regional effect of monosodium-L-glutamate on the superficial layers of superior colliculus in rat." *Cell Tissue Res* 235 (2): 453–7.

Shao Z, Rompe G, Schiltenwolf M. 2002. "Radiographic changes in the lumbar intervertebral discs and lumbar vertebrae with age." *Spine* 27 (February 1): 263–8.

Sindrup SH, Jensen TS. 1999. "Efficacy of pharmacological treatments of neuropathic pain: an update and effect related to mechanis, of drug action." *Pain* 83 (December): 389–400.

Singer, B., Ryff, C. D., & Seeman, T. 2004. "Operationalizing Allostatic Load." In J. Schulkin (Ed.), Allostasis, Homeostasis, and the Costs of Physiological Adaptation. Cambridge: Cambridge University Press.

Slosberg M. 2009. "Essentials of Dynamic Stability Training and Chiropractic Care." *Dyn Chiro* 27(2):1-5.

Smith JC. 2014. "Climbing the ladder of opportunity—the death knell of spine surgery and the opportunity for doctors of chiropractic to ascend the health care ladder." *Dynamic Chiropractic* 32(06):1-9.

Söderholm JD, Perdue MH. 2001. "Stress and gastrointestinal tract. II. Stress and intestinal barrier function." *Am J Physiol Gastrointest Liver Physiol* 280 (January): G7–G13.

Sterling, P. 2004 "Principles of allostasis: optimal design, predictive regulation, pathophysiology and rational therapeutics." In J. Schulkin (Ed.), Allostasis, Homeostasis, and the Costs of Physiological Adaptation. Cambridge: Cambridge University Press.

Sztajzel J. 2004. "Heart rate variability: a noninvasive electrocardiographic method to measure the autonomic nervous system." *Swiss Medical Weekly* 134 (September): 514–22.

Taylor MK, et al. 2007. "Neurophysiologic methods to measure stress during survival, evasion, resistance, and escape training." *Aviation, Space, & Environmental Medicine* 78 (May): B224–30.

Thompson DG, Richelson E, Malagelada JR. 1982. "Perturbation of gastric emptying and duodenal motility through the central nervous system." *Gastroenterology* 83 (December): 1200–6.

Thompson DG, Richelson E, Malagelada JR. 1983. "Perturbation of upper gastrointestinal function by cold stress." *Gut* 24 (April): 277–83.

Timmins, William G. 2011. *The Chronic Stress Crisis*. Bloomington: AuthorHouse.

Tsao H, Danneels LA, Hodges PW. 2011. "ISSLS prize winners: Smudging the motor brain in young adults with recurrent low back pain." *Spine* 26 (October 1): 1721–7.

Tumminello, N. 2012. "The cause of low back pain: New science questions conventional wisdom surrounding this common affliction." (September 7) accessed at **www.livestrong.com**

Turnbaugh, Peter J., et al. 2009. "The Effect of Diet on the Human Gut Microbiome: A Metagenomic Analysis in Humanized Gnotobiotic Mice." *Science Translational Medicine* 1 (November): 6ra14.

Twomey L, Taylor JR. 1985. "Age changes in lumbar intervertebral discs." *Acta Orthop Scand* 56: 496–499.

Urquhart DM, Hodges PW. 2005. "Differential activity of regions of trans- versus abdominis during trunk rotation." *Eur Spine J* 14: 393–400.

Vallfors B.1985. Acute, Subacute and Chronic Low Back Pain: Clinical Symptoms, Absenteeism and Working Environment. *Scan J Rehab Med Suppl* 11: 1-98.

Van Tulder MW, Touray T, Furlan AD, Solway S, Bouter LM. 2003. "Muscle relaxants for nonspecific low back pain: a systematic review within the framework of the cochrane collaboration." *Spine* 28 (September 1): 1978–92.

Vegfors M, Tryggvason B, Sjöberg F, Lennmarken C. 1990. "Assessment of peripheral blood flow using a pulse oximeter." *Journal of Clinical Monitoring* 6 (January): 1–4.

Vgontzas AN, et al. 1999. "Sleep deprivation effects on the activity of the hypothalamic-pituitary-adrenal and growth axes: potential clinical implications." *Clin Endocrinol (Oxf)* 51 (August): 205–15.

Vgontzas AN, Chrousos GP. 2002. "Sleep, the hypothalamic-pituitary-adrenal axis, and cytokines: multiple interactions and disturbances in sleep disorders." *Endocrinol Metab Clin North Am.* 31 (March): 15–36.

Walker AW, Lawley TD. 2013. "Therapeutic modulation of intestinal dysbiosis." *Pharmacology Research* 69 (March): 75–86.

Watson CP. 2000. "The treatment of neuropathic pain: antidepressants and opioids." *Clin J Pain* 16 (2 supp): S49–S55.

Waris E, Eskelin M, Hermunen H, Kiviluoto O, Paajanen H. 2007. "Disc degeneration in low back pain: a 17-year follow-up study using magnetic resonance imaging." *Spine* 32 (March 15): 681–4.

Weil, Andrew. 2005. *Mind Body Tool Kit.* Boulder: Body & Soul Onmimedia.

Weiniger, Stephen P. 2008. *Stand Taller ~ Live Longer: An Anti-Aging Strategy.* Alpharetta: BodyZone.

Wheeler AH, Murrey DB. 2005. *Spinal pain: pathogenesis, evolutionary mechanisms, and management, in Pappagallo M (ed). The neurological basis of pain.* New York: McGraw-Hill: 421-52.

Wheeler A. 2009. "Lowback pain and sciatica: pathogenesis, diagnosis, and nonoperative treatment." In *Practical Guides to Chronic Pain Syndromes,* edited by G. Jay, 181–204. New York: Informa.

Williams CL, Peterson JM, Villar RG, Burks TF. 1987. "Corticotropin-releasing factor directly mediates colonic responses to stress." *American Journal of Physiology* 253 (October): G582–6.

Wolf, Robb. 2010. *The Paleo Solution: The Original Human Diet.* Las Vegas: Victory Belt.

Wood, Alex M., et al. 2009. "Gratitude influences sleep through the mechanism of pre-sleep cognitions." *Journal of Psychosomatic Research* 66: 43–48.

Yamazaki H, Nishiyama J, Suzuki T. 2012. "Use of perfusion index from pulse oximetry to determine efficacy of stellate ganglion block." *Local & Regional Anesthesia* 5: 9–14.

Zareie M, et al. 2006. "Probiotics prevent bacterial translocation and improve intestinal barrier function in rats following chronic psychological stress." *Gut* 55 (November): 1553–1560.

Zhao CQ, Wang LM, Jiang LS, Dai LY. 2007. "The cell biology of intervertebral disc aging and degeneration." *Ageing Res Rev* 6 (October): 247–61. Epub 2007 (August 10).

www.ingramcontent.com/pod-product-compliance
Lightning Source LLC
Chambersburg PA
CBHW030418290526
45786CB00001B/36